Faith Prevailed

A Testimony of God's Faithfulness in the
Journey of Infertility
Kemi Adetola

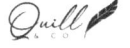

Quill and Company

ISBN: 979-8-9925856-6-7

Published by: Quill & Company Publishing
thequillandcompany@gmail.com

First edition, 2025
Printed in the United States of America

Contents

To God Almighty, the Alpha and Omega —You were our anchor in the storm, the source of our enduring hope, and the provider of the miracle we now hold close. We dedicate this testimony to Your unfailing love and perfect timing.

To our precious twins, Tobi and Tomi—your vibrant lives are a living testament that God is always on time, never early, never late. You are the long-awaited melody that fills our home with joy and reminds us of answered prayers.

To every couple still navigating the challenging path of waiting—may our story serve as a beacon of hope, a reminder that a delay is never a denial, and that God continues to pen the most beautiful and unexpected narratives.

"But those who wait upon the Lord shall renew their strength; they shall mount up with wings like eagles, they shall run and not be weary, they shall walk and not faint."

- Isaiah 40:31 (NKJV)

Preface
WHERE CULTURE MEETS CALLING

I am a proud Yoruba man, rooted deeply in Nigerian culture—a heritage that reveres family, community, and the continuity of legacy above all else. In our society, the arrival of a child soon after marriage isn't merely anticipated; it's an expectation, almost a mandate. Parenthood is seen as a profound mark of honor, validating both manhood and womanhood. Consequently, a couple who remains childless often becomes the subject of whispers. These whispers can quickly escalate into direct questions, which then morph into intense pressure, ultimately breeding a profound sense of shame.

For two decades, my wife and I found ourselves living under the weight of this cultural expectation. The messages, though often unsaid directly, were unmistakably clear. Some would gently suggest adoption, while others subtly hinted at the idea of remarriage. The judgment sometimes came cloaked in sarcasm: "Don't you want to become a man yet?" Others ventured into spiritual assumptions, questioning if our prayers or fasts were sufficient, or implying hidden sin.

My heart ached most for my wife, Kemi. In our culture, the woman often bears the heaviest burden of infertility, even when the cause is unknown or shared. She was treated differently, subjected to comments no one has a right to utter. As rich and beautiful as our Yoruba culture is, it undeniably has its imperfections. When it comes to infertility, these flaws can become sharp instruments, even within the confines of the church. This unfortunate reality explains why so many marriages falter and crumble under the immense weight of childlessness. Some men, tragically, choose the "Abraham route," introducing another wife into the marital equation. Yet, much like in biblical accounts, such decisions rarely end well. Polygamy inevitably ushers in jealousy, envy, and conflict, tearing homes apart and diverting destinies—all because societal pressure proved too overwhelming for both community and couple.

There's a popular saying in the business world: "Culture will eat strategy for breakfast." I've come to believe this isn't just true in business; it's devastatingly accurate in the context of marriage. Many couples begin their journey with pure intentions, faithfully praying, exploring medical options, and holding onto hope. However, their communities, churches, and even close friends can unwittingly act as spiritual saboteurs, inadvertently twisting genuine faith into fanaticism and demonizing valid medical science. One of the most heartbreaking realities I've witnessed is how Christians, who should embody compassion, often display the most closed-mindedness when it comes to fertility treatments or surrogacy. Some dismiss surrogacy entirely without truly understanding it, leading many couples to miss their opportune moment and later live with the quiet pain of profound regret.

My own perspective underwent a profound shift when my wife—steadfast and remarkably wise—gently reminded me: "Even Jesus came through surrogacy. Mary carried Him, but the seed wasn't from Joseph." That singular truth revolutionized my understanding. God possesses the power to bring forth life in any manner He chooses. If He could part the Red Sea, He is certainly capable of opening a womb. If He could open Sarah's womb in her old age, He can undoubtedly open doors through the advancements of modern medicine. Miracles, we've learned, are not always mystical; often, they are medical. We are living proof of this profound truth.

This book is more than just our personal narrative; it is intended as a lifeline for couples battling infertility in silence. If you are advancing in age, consider preserving your embryos. If you feel weary, dedicate yourselves to strengthening both your faith and your practical strategy. Most importantly, surround yourselves with individuals who are informed, compassionate, and firmly rooted in truth, rather than solely in rigid tradition. Because on this arduous journey, it is not only the heart that must remain strong, but also the mind.

To all who continue to wait: *God is still meticulously writing your unique story. Do not close the book prematurely. Faith will prevail.*

— *Yemi Adetola*

Introduction

THE CALL THAT CHANGED EVERYTHING

I remember the moment as if it were etched in time, a single frame suspended in the reel of my memory. It was a Saturday morning, April 1, 2023, a day that began with the mundane rhythm of weekend errands. The air held the promise of a simple, ordinary day. My husband and I were on our way to the gym, a routine we cherished, but decided to make a quick stop at Sam's Club first. As we sat in the parking lot, bathed in the ordinary morning light, my phone buzzed. The sound was unremarkable, a familiar vibration against the console, but the text it announced was from my doctor in Nigeria. My heart leaped into my throat, a frantic, hopeful drumbeat against my ribs. My hands were shaking so much I could barely hold the phone steady, the screen a blur of my own anxious reflection. I took a deep, shuddering breath and read the words that would unravel nineteen years of pain and change my life forever:

"Congratulations, your gestational carrier is pregnant."

I was confused. I was shocked. I read the words again, and then a third time, my mind struggling to grasp their meaning. Is this for real? The date, April 1st, flashed in my mind—a cruel, cosmic joke? But the words on the screen were clear, unwavering. I was in the car with my husband when I got the text, and a sound escaped my lips, half-sob, half-shout of disbelief. I just burst out crying. The tears I had shed for nineteen years—tears of grief, of frustration, of a hope that had worn thin—were suddenly replaced by a torrent of a different kind. I couldn't believe it was true. After nineteen years of waiting, of praying, of hoping, of a silence in our home that had become deafening, it was finally, impossibly, happening. We were pregnant.

We went into Sam's Club, but I don't think we bought a single thing. We were moving through a world that suddenly felt different, as if we were encased in a bubble of joy and disbelief. The towering shelves of bulk goods, the bright fluorescent lights, the hum of other families going about their day—it all felt like a movie playing in the background of our own surreal, beautiful scene. I had to compose myself, to try to act normal, but inside, I was exploding with a joy so immense it felt like it was going to burst out of me. We wandered the aisles, aimlessly pushing an empty cart, looking at each other every few minutes and bursting into uncontrollable laughter. We left the store and just sat in the car for a moment, the engine off, letting the monumental reality of the news sink into the quiet space between us.

Later that evening, the joy still electric in the air, I called my friends—Abiodun (Abbey), Ebere, and Ram—to let them know. With each call, the miracle felt more real, the words "we're pregnant" solidifying from a dream into a tangible truth. Their voices, filled with the same unadulterated joy and excitement that I was feeling, were a beautiful echo of our own. It was a day of celebration, a day of answered prayers, a day the Lord had truly made.

I want to encourage couples who are struggling with infertility to not give up, to be consistent. That's one thing I learned in my own story: I was consistent. I did not give up, even when everything—my body, my emotions, the passing of time—seemed to be against me. I knew, one way or another, that I was going to have children. I had frozen embryos, precious sparks of hope stored away, and I was determined to see them have a chance at life. The truth is, I was shocked when the pregnancy news came because a part of me had become so accustomed to disappointment. But I was just doing what I knew I had to do, taking the next step of faith, and then the next. I want to encourage couples to be open to the options that God has given us through doctors and the science of infertility treatment. People prayed for me at retreats, at prayer sessions, and I am so deeply grateful for their support, which was a lifeline in my darkest hours.

Infertility is a journey marked by profound emotional, physical, and spiritual challenges. When you have trusted God for so long for children, you would think people would be sensitive, but that wasn't always my story. This is a testimony of resilience, faith, and the unwavering, often mysterious, love of God.

My husband and I got married on September 7, 2002. Our journey into the world of infertility began with visiting five clinics and starting fertility treatments in 2005. The hope that each new treatment brought was a fragile, beautiful thing, a delicate flame that was repeatedly extinguished by the cold wind of a negative result. After 21 years of marriage and 19 years of longing for a child, God remained faithful to my husband and me. He blessed us with twins in 2023. Each step of the way, God's timing and love were evident, reminding us of Isaiah 40:31: "But those who trust in the Lord will find new strength. They will soar high on wings like eagles. They will run and not grow weary. They will walk and not faint."

From My Husband's Perspective:

I never imagined that becoming a father would take 21 years.

When my wife and I got married, we had dreams—vivid, hopeful dreams—of building a home filled with love, laughter, and the chaotic, beautiful sound of children's feet running through the halls. But year after year, those halls remained quiet. The silence was a presence in itself, a constant reminder of what was missing. We tried to stay hopeful. We smiled when others celebrated births, a smile that often masked a deep, piercing ache. We prayed. We waited. We believed.

For 19 years, we pursued every possible path—IUI, IVF, and finally, surrogacy. We sat in countless waiting rooms, the air thick with unspoken hopes and fears, a silent camaraderie with the other couples who shared our journey. We endured procedures and setbacks, each one chipping away at our reserves of strength and hope. We wrestled with a profound silence from heaven and the relentless noise from the world around us: the questions, the assumptions, the well-meaning but often hurtful advice, and even the judgments. Behind every smile I wore in public was a private grief, the quiet sorrow of a man expected to be a pillar of strength for his wife. I was the husband—often expected to be strong, always trying to be hopeful—but sometimes, I was simply hurting.

Still, I held on to my faith. Not because I always felt strong, but because I had nowhere else to go. I clung to God, even when His timing didn't make sense, even when my own prayers felt like they were hitting a brass ceiling. My wife and I walked through this valley together—sometimes with tears, sometimes in a silence born of a shared pain too deep for words—but always with a shared, unspoken determination: we would not give up.

And then... the miracle came. Not in the way we had so meticulously planned or desperately prayed for. But in God's perfect, extravagant timing, through the gift of surrogacy, our twins were born. Healthy. Beautiful. They were worth every tear, every test, every year of waiting. Every single moment of pain was redeemed in the instant I held them in my arms.

In this book, I add my perspective as a husband—a man of faith navigating the long, arduous, and often lonely road of infertility, marriage, and fatherhood. It's a testimony to the power of persistence, the strength of a love tested by fire, and the boundless grace of God.

Because through it all, no matter how long it took... faith prevailed.

Our story is a testament to the fact that God's plans are not our plans, and His ways are not our ways. We began our journey with a simple, human-sized dream, and He ended it with a miracle that was far beyond anything we could have ever imagined. This book is the story of that journey, a journey that took us through the depths of despair and to the heights of a joy so profound it still takes my breath away.

In the chapters that follow, we will invite you into our story. We will take you with us into the sterile waiting rooms, into the tense operating rooms, and into the quiet, sacred spaces where we wrestled with God and with each other. We will not shy away from the raw, honest details of our struggle—the physical pain of the procedures, the emotional toll of the disappointments, the spiritual battles we fought against doubt and despair. We will pull back the curtain on the cultural pressures that threatened to crush us, the insensitive comments that wounded us, and the incredible community of friends and family that ultimately carried us.

We will also share the moments of breathtaking grace, the glimmers of hope that sustained us in the darkness. We will tell you about the prophetic baby shower that spoke of twins seventeen years before they arrived, the unwavering support of our prayer partners who held up our arms when we were too weak to stand, and the miraculous provision of our community that turned an impossible dream into a reality. We will take you on the surreal, anxiety-ridden journey of shipping our precious embryos across an ocean, and we will let you experience the heart-stopping moment when we learned that after nineteen years of barrenness, we were finally, miraculously, pregnant with twins.

This is a story about the messy, complicated, and beautiful reality of a faith that is lived out in the real world. It's a story about a marriage that was tested by fire and came out stronger, more resilient, and more deeply in love on the other side. It's a story about a God who is not afraid of our questions, our anger, or our doubt, a God who meets us in our brokenness and, in His perfect, unhurried time, turns our mourning into dancing.

Our prayer is that this book will be a source of hope and encouragement for all who read it. If you are in the midst of your own journey of infertility, we want you to know that you are not alone. We see you, we understand your pain, and we are praying for you. And if you are a friend or family member of someone walking this road, we pray our story offers you a window into their world, equipping you with the understanding and compassion needed to be a true source of support and grace.

This is not just our story; it is a story of God's faithfulness. The chapters that follow serve as our testament, establishing the core themes of the book and chronicling the incredible journey that brought us our children and taught us the true meaning of faith.

Chapter 1
THE WEDDING AND THE WAITING

Before my husband and I got married, we sat down and had one of those earnest, hope-filled conversations that young, in-love couples have, mapping out a future that seemed so clear and straightforward it felt like simple arithmetic. We were cocooned in the blissful certainty that our love, combined with a sensible plan, was all we needed. We agreed, with the easy confidence of youth, that we would wait two years before starting a family. It felt like a wise, responsible decision, a testament to our maturity. We wanted time to build our foundation as a couple, to grow in our careers, to simply enjoy the quiet intimacy and shared laughter of being husband and wife before welcoming children into our lives. We stepped into our marriage on September 7, 2002, armed with a practical plan, a clear timeline, and a heart full of unblemished dreams.

It took less than a month for the pressure to begin.

In our Nigerian culture, especially within the Yoruba community, a marriage is not just a union of two people; it is a covenant between two families, a public institution with the expectation of continuing a lineage. The birth of a child is the immediate, expected seal on that covenant, the tangible proof that the union is blessed and fruitful. The questions started almost instantly, not with malice, but with an ingrained cultural expectancy that felt as natural and necessary as breathing to those around us. An auntie would pull me aside at a bustling family function, her eyes sparkling with a mixture of genuine affection and pointed curiosity, and ask, "So, Kemi, any news for us?" At church, a well-meaning elder would pat my stomach, a gesture both kind and profoundly invasive, and say with a knowing smile, "We are praying for you! Very soon!" It was a constant, public monitoring of my womb, my body treated as a communal project. It was a bizarre and unsettling feeling. At first, it was easy to laugh it off, to deflect with a smile. "Not yet, Auntie! We are still enjoying being married!" But as the months turned into a year, then two, the tone shifted. The questions became more pointed, the smiles tinged with a subtle, sorrowful pity. The clock was ticking, and it felt like our entire community was listening.

The pressure came from all sides, a chorus of voices telling me what I should be doing. "You better hurry up," one person advised, their words a painful, constant reminder of my own biological clock. "A man can have kids at any age, but a woman's time is short." The implication was clear and sharp: I was falling behind, and my husband had options that I did not. People began to blame me silently, their assumptions hanging heavy and suffocating in the air. I would walk into a room, and the conversation would drop to a whisper, resuming only after I had passed. I could feel their eyes on me, their unspoken thoughts a palpable weight. Why isn't she pregnant yet? Is something wrong with her?

From My Husband's Perspective:

I saw the pressure building on Kemi, and it was hard to watch the light in her eyes dim with each passing month. I tried to shield her as best I could, to be a buffer against the world's relentless expectations. When relatives would corner me, their questions disguised as concern, I would politely but firmly tell them, "We have a plan. We will have children in God's time." I wanted them to know that we were a team, that this was our decision, our journey, not just hers to bear alone. But the cultural weight was immense, a relentless tide. It was a constant battle to protect her from the well-meaning but often hurtful intrusions of our community, a community we loved but that didn't understand the private battle we were beginning to wage.

Kemi's Perspective:

The emotional toll was immense. Social gatherings, once a source of joy, became minefields of potential pain. There were times I just didn't feel like going out. I would decline invitations to birthday parties or baby showers because the effort of putting on a brave face, of celebrating a joy that felt so impossibly far from my own, was simply too exhausting. The performance of happiness was a weight too heavy to bear. My husband would find me on the sofa, quiet and withdrawn, the unspoken sadness a third presence in the room, and he would know. "We don't have to go," he'd say gently, his hand on my shoulder. But I knew that hiding away wasn't a solution. I just didn't know how to navigate the pain.

I found myself in a constant, running conversation with God, my prayers a tangled web of confusion and frustration. "God, what is all this? Why is this happening? I thought we were following your will." The journey was already painful, a landscape of quiet sorrow and unanswered questions, and we hadn't even begun to face the medical challenges that lay ahead.

By 2005, our two-year plan had come and gone, and my womb was still empty. The pressure, both internal and external, had become unbearable. We decided it was time to seek medical help. In May of that year, I started my first IUI treatment. I was so hopeful, clinging to the promise of science as a lifeline. This, I thought, would be the answer. The science would solve the problem. But it failed. And so began a new chapter in our journey, a grueling cycle of hope and despair that would define our lives for years to come. I tried another IUI, and then another. We moved from a clinic in Rockville to one in Virginia, searching for a different doctor, a different protocol, a different result. But the answer was always the same: a stark, clinical, soul-crushing negative.

With each failed cycle, the emotional weight grew heavier. The process itself was a logistical and emotional marathon. I was a working woman, building a career, and yet my life was dictated by ovulation cycles and clinic appointments. I would have to get up in the dark, before the sun rose, to drive to my appointments, battling rush hour traffic to get there on time so I could get back for a full day of work. I remember the exhaustion, the profound feeling of living a double life—the competent, smiling professional on the outside, and the heartbroken, struggling woman on the inside.

This is when the support of my community became a true lifeline. I thank God every day for my immediate family, my friends, and my siblings, who were my rock. They never wavered in their support, never questioned our decisions. They were just there, a constant, loving presence in the storm.

And then there were my friends. My dear friend Abiodun, whom I call Abbey, was my prayer partner through it all. She stayed with me through every high and every crushing low. She was the one I would call from the car, my voice choked with tears after another negative result, unable to even form the words. She wouldn't offer easy platitudes or simple solutions; she would just listen, creating a sacred space in the silence for my grief. And then she would pray, her faith a shield when my own was riddled with holes. I thank God for her support and encouragement. It was a gift of immeasurable worth.

I also clung to the promises of God. I stood on the belief that He would not fail me. I committed myself to the truth that His promises are "yes and amen." My faith was not in the doctors or the treatments; it was in my God. But I was beginning to understand that this journey was also a battle. It was a spiritual fight, and I needed to be strong. The depression that can accompany infertility is real and it is dark, a heavy fog that threatens to obscure all light. I needed every ounce of strength I could muster to keep from sinking into its depths. The journey was long, and I was just at the beginning.

As the years of failed IUIs stacked up, the whispers from the community grew louder and more pointed. It felt as though my value as a woman was being questioned, not just by others, but sometimes, in my darkest moments, by myself. The feeling of inadequacy was a constant, unwelcome companion, a shadow that followed me everywhere. I felt like I was failing at the most fundamental aspect of womanhood. Some people, and the devil himself, made me feel like I had failed as a woman, that I was somehow incomplete. The hurtful comments from those who didn't understand our struggle compounded my pain. They whispered that I should have started trying earlier, that maybe, somehow, this was all my fault. These judgments were daggers to my heart, deepening a sorrow that already felt bottomless.

Mother's Day became a particularly painful reminder of what I longed for and had not yet achieved. Every year, it was a day of deep, profound sorrow, not only because of my own empty arms but also because I lost my mother in March of

2012. The grief of her absence, a raw and open wound, combined with my own struggles with infertility, made Mother's Day an incredibly difficult time. My mother had been my biggest cheerleader, my fiercest advocate. She was the one who believed, with every fiber of her being, that I would one day hold my own child. Her passing left a void that felt especially vast on that particular Sunday in May.

To make matters worse, there was a particular woman who, every year, would find a way to twist the knife. Instead of a simple "Happy Mother's Day," a greeting extended to all women in our culture as a sign of respect, she would say something like, "I will wish you a happy Mother's Day once you have kids." I can't imagine what would possess someone to say something so deliberately cruel. You don't have to have biological children to be wished a Happy Mother's Day. Her words were a deliberate denial of my worth, a public declaration that, in her eyes, I was not yet complete. How could someone weaponize a day of honor? It affected me deeply, year after year.

The spiritual pressure was just as intense. People would randomly approach me in church and start praying, laying hands on my stomach without my permission. I didn't have any relationship with these individuals, and their public displays of "concern" only made me feel more like a spectacle, more inadequate in my faith. The situation was made even more challenging when people would compare my spirituality unfavorably to my husband's, especially after yet another failed IVF cycle. "Maybe his faith is stronger than yours," someone once suggested, a comment that was devastatingly painful and planted seeds of doubt.

People also began to invite me to visit other churches, assuming my infertility was the result of a curse that my own church wasn't powerful enough to break. Some asked me to visit a prophet in South Africa. Others suggested seeking out a prophet in the mountains. I am so grateful that, because of my deep trust in God, these people didn't sway me to follow their advice. I knew God had already answered my prayers. I was in a season of thanksgiving, choosing to praise God in spite of all the negative comments and the disappointing results.

But despite the critics, there were many friends who came alongside us in praying and believing for children. In 2006, a few friends from my church surprised me with a faith-filled baby shower. I will never forget how one particular friend actually bought clothes for twins—a boy and a girl. They prayed and encouraged me that my time would surely come. Their faith was a beacon in the darkness, a tangible expression of a hope I was struggling to hold onto.

After several years of failed IUIs, the doctors recommended we move on to IVF. This was a whole new level of physical, emotional, and financial commitment. The IVF process was grueling. It was a constant cycle of medications, injections, and monitoring appointments, all of which I had to manage while working a demanding full-time job. I would wake up in the pre-dawn darkness to beat the traffic, driving to clinics in Virginia, Maryland, and Washington D.C., and then rush to work, trying to act as if my morning hadn't been filled with invasive procedures and anxious waiting. The emotional toll after each consultation, especially after a failed cycle, was devastating.

In this journey, I experienced the heartbreak of two chemical pregnancies, a ghost of a hope that was whispered and then snatched away. And I lost both of my fallopian tubes to an infection, a loss that required major surgery and a painful recovery. This was a point of no return, a surgical finality that closed the door on a natural pregnancy forever. Through all of these devastating losses, my friend Abbey, my prayer partner, was my constant support. My community stood by me. They loaned me their faith when mine faltered, and their prayers held me up in an extremely difficult time. We also used our own faith to encourage others going through similar battles. I remember advising one couple to pursue a gestational carrier, sharing the little I knew, and they followed our advice. Later, we found out they had children, and we were thrilled that our guidance had led to such a positive outcome. But still, we were waiting for our own miracle.

I held onto my faith, and I had hope against hope that God would come through for us. I hung onto prophecies from pastors, friends, and family members about us having children. I wasn't sure how it would happen, especially after I lost my fallopian tubes, but I trusted God. I had heard stories of supernatural miracles where people had children even without a uterus. I knew that many people were praying for us, and that encouraged me. I drew strength from Exodus 23:26, where God promises the Israelites that "none will miscarry or be barren in the land." I believed that we would have children—it was only a matter of time.

Prayer Point:

Heavenly Father, thank You for the beautiful gift of marriage and the dreams You place in our hearts. As we begin this journey, shield our hearts from the pressure of timelines and the weight of outside expectations. May Your voice be the loudest we hear, and grant us the patience to trust Your perfect timing, even when the waiting begins. Protect our bond and let us find our strength in You and in each other. Amen.

Chapter 2
The First Steps

By the beginning of 2005, the quiet ache of waiting had become a constant, undeniable presence in my life. We had been married for nearly three years, and the imaginary window of our "two-year plan" had firmly, audibly, clicked shut. The pressure from our community was relentless, a steady hum of expectation in the background of our lives. But the pressure from within my own heart was even greater, a silent scream that no one else could hear. I had longed to be a mother for as long as I could remember, and the continued absence of a child felt like a fundamental piece of me was missing, a hollow space where a life was meant to be. From January to May of that year, I tracked my cycles with a growing sense of dread. Each month was a fresh cycle of hope and loss. Nothing was happening. It was clear that we needed to do something more than just hope and pray. Action was required.

It was my idea to seek medical help, a suggestion I made with a lump in my throat. My husband, ever supportive, agreed immediately. He could see the toll the waiting was taking on me, the way the light in my eyes dimmed a little more with each passing month. He was ready to face whatever came next, as long as we faced it together. I made an appointment with my primary care doctor, who listened with a deep and genuine compassion before giving me a referral to a fertility clinic in Rockville, Maryland. That slip of paper felt like a key, a tangible object that could unlock a door to a new world of possibility. I called the clinic that day and scheduled our first appointment, my voice trembling slightly as I spoke the words aloud.

I remember walking into that clinic for the first time, a bundle of raw nerves and fragile, carefully guarded hope. The waiting room was sterile and quiet, the air thick with unspoken anxieties. It was filled with other couples who all wore the same strained expression, a mask of forced calm that I recognized instantly. To be honest, I was very shy. The process felt so incredibly private, and I was acutely, painfully aware that by being there, I was making a public declaration of our struggle. I didn't want people to know my business. I didn't want to be the subject of gossip or pity. But I knew this was a necessary step.

The first consultation was a whirlwind of information, a dizzying onslaught of medical terms and possibilities. We met with a doctor who walked us through the initial diagnostic process. They took my blood to check my hormone levels, all of which came back normal. This was both a relief and a profound source of frustration. If nothing was wrong, why wasn't I getting pregnant? The nurses then explained the first course of action they recommended: Intrauterine Insemination, or IUI.

They explained that I would take medication to stimulate my ovaries to produce multiple eggs. Then, at the precise time of ovulation, they would take a prepared sample of my husband's sperm and, using a thin catheter, place it directly into my uterus to give it the best possible chance of reaching the egg. It sounded so scientific, so logical, so full of promise. For the first time in years, I felt a surge of real, tangible hope. This was a plan. This was action. We were no longer just waiting; we were fighting.

And so began the cycle that would come to define our lives for years to come. The first part of the IUI process was a flurry of activity. I was prescribed medication to stimulate egg production. This was followed by frequent, early-morning visits to the clinic for bloodwork and ultrasounds to monitor the growth of the follicles. Each visit was filled with a nervous anticipation that bordered on terror. Were the medications working? Were the follicles growing? Every positive sign was a small, hard-won victory, a reason to let a little more hope seep in.

Then came the day of the procedure itself. It was quick and relatively painless, but emotionally, it was monumental. As I lay on the table, the sterile lights of the procedure room shining down, I prayed with every fiber of my being. "Lord, let this be it. Please, let this be the time."

And then came the hardest part of all: the two-week wait.

For two weeks, my life was a state of suspended animation. Every twinge, every cramp, every fleeting wave of nausea was a potential sign, a whisper of a promise. I was caught in a constant, dizzying cycle of hope and fear. One moment, I would be mentally planning the nursery in my head, imagining the moment the doctor would call with good news. The next, the crushing fear of another disappointment would wash over me, so potent it felt hard to breathe. I was desperate for it to work.

Finally, the day of the blood test arrived. I went to the clinic, my heart pounding with a mixture of hope and dread. Then, I went home to wait for the call. When the phone rang, I snatched it up, my hand trembling.

"I'm sorry, Kemi," the nurse said, her voice laced with a practiced compassion that did little to soften the blow. "The test was negative."

The word hit me with the force of a physical blow. Negative. I couldn't believe it. I was so sure this time. I had felt pregnant. The hope that had sustained me for two weeks evaporated in an instant, replaced by a grief so deep it felt like I was drowning. I cried, deep, wracking sobs that seemed to come from the very core of my being. I was devastated.

From My Husband's Perspective:

I was shocked. In my mind, this was supposed to be the answer. I never thought that we would go through all of this just for it to fail. I had watched Kemi endure the medications and the appointments, and I was so hopeful for her. To see her so completely devastated was heartbreaking. It was a brutal introduction to the reality that medical science was not a magic wand. It was just another path filled with uncertainty. I didn't know what to do or say to comfort her. I just held her, my own heart aching with a profound sense of helplessness. This was a shock to our system, a loss that we both felt deeply, but in different ways.

The pain of that first negative result was immense. I had thought the experience would be easy, that the doctors would have a simple solution. The reality was so much more painful than I could have imagined. I was down, but I was not out. My hope was bruised, but it was not broken. After the tears had dried, a familiar feeling rose up within me: determination. I was consistent. I did not give up. I knew, with a certainty that defied my circumstances, that this was just the beginning. There would be more attempts. This was just the first step on a long road, and I was ready to keep walking.

Kemi's Perspective:

The aftermath of that first failed IUI was a desolate landscape. My husband was in a state of shock. He had always believed that we would get pregnant naturally, and the idea of needing medical assistance was something he had struggled to accept. In his mind, this first attempt was supposed to be a quick fix, a simple solution to a temporary problem. The negative result was a brutal awakening, a sudden, jarring realization that our path was not going to be as straightforward as he had imagined. The pain of it all hit him hard, and seeing his own hope crumble was another layer of sorrow for me to bear.

I, on the other hand, had a different reaction. The initial devastation gave way to a familiar resolve. I had been living with the weight of this struggle for years, and while the disappointment was acute, it did not extinguish the fire in my spirit. I went to the crate where I kept my Bible and my journals, and I just opened them up, searching for solace, for guidance, for a reason to keep going. I turned on some worship music, letting the songs of faith wash over me, a balm to my wounded soul. I prayed, not with the desperate hope of the two-week wait, but with a quiet, steely determination. "Okay, God," I said, "this is just the beginning. I know there will be many more attempts. So be it. I'm not giving up."

And so began the cycle that would define our lives for the next several years. We tried another IUI, and another, and another. Each one was a miniature lifetime compressed into a few short weeks. It started with the hopeful anticipation of a new cycle, the diligent administration of medications, the frequent trips to the clinic. It peaked with the tense, prayer-filled moment of the procedure itself. Then came the agonizing two-week wait, a tightrope walk between hope and despair. And finally, it would end with the crushing finality of another negative result.

With each failure, the emotional toll mounted. The initial, bright-eyed hope of that first cycle was replaced by a more cautious, guarded optimism. We learned to protect our hearts, to not let ourselves get too excited. But no matter how much you try, the hope is always there, a stubborn little flame that refuses to be extinguished. And when the negative result came again, it burned just as badly.

The financial strain also began to take its toll. Each IUI cycle cost thousands of dollars, and the bills were piling up. We were pouring our savings into a dream that seemed to be slipping further and further away. The stress of it all began to seep into every corner of our lives, creating a tension that was always present, just beneath the surface.

From My Husband's Perspective:

With each failed attempt, I felt a growing sense of frustration and anger. I was angry at the situation, angry at the unfairness of it all. I saw other couples getting pregnant with ease, some who didn't even seem to want children, and I would ask God, "Why them and not us?" It was hard to see Kemi go through the physical and emotional rollercoaster each month, and I often didn't know what to say. I would just try to be strong for her, to be a source of constant encouragement, even when I was struggling with my own doubts and disappointments.

My private conversations with God during this time were a raw mixture of prayer, praise, and desperate pleading. I would listen to worship songs, trying to fill my heart with hope and drown out the whispers of doubt. I thanked God for getting us this far, for giving us access to medical help. I thanked Him for the small signs of progress, for the support of our family and friends. But I also cried out to Him in my confusion and pain. "God, why is this so hard? What do you want me to do?" I just needed His guidance. I felt like I was walking in the dark, and I desperately needed Him to light the path ahead.

Kemi's Perspective:

It was during this time that I truly began to understand the power of my community. My friend Abbey was my constant prayer warrior. She would check in with me throughout each cycle, sending me scriptures and words of encouragement. When a cycle failed, she would mourn with me, her empathy a soothing balm to my wounded spirit. Her steadfast support was a tangible expression of God's love, a reminder that I was not alone in my struggle.

After several failed IUIs at the clinic in Rockville, we decided it was time for a change. We moved to a new clinic in Virginia, hoping that a different doctor, a different approach, might yield a different result. But the story remained the same. Cycle after cycle ended in disappointment.

The cumulative effect of these repeated failures was profound. My initial shyness about the process had been replaced by a weary resignation. My body felt like a science experiment, poked and prodded and measured, but ultimately, failing to perform. The hope that had once been a blazing fire had been reduced to a fragile ember, one that I had to fight to keep from being extinguished completely.

But even in the midst of the disappointment, my faith, though tested, did not break. I was consistent. I did not give up. I drew strength from the promises of God, from the love of my husband, and from the unwavering support of my community. I knew, with a certainty that defied my circumstances, that our story was not over. This was just one chapter. And as this chapter of failed IUIs came to a close, I knew we were on the cusp of a new one. The doctors were beginning to whisper a new set of letters, a new, more intensive path: IVF. It was a daunting prospect, but I was ready. I would do whatever it took to hold my baby in my arms. The journey was long, but my resolve was strong. Faith, I was learning, was not about avoiding the valley; it was about walking through it, one step at a time, with your eyes fixed on the hope that lies on the other side.

Prayer Point:

Lord, give us the strength to endure and the grace to hope again. Let Your voice be louder than the silence we hear each month. Fill our hearts with peace, and remind us that You are with us—even when nothing makes sense. In Jesus' name, Amen.

Chapter 3
THE ESCALATION TO IVF

After the repeated failures of the IUI cycles, a heavy sense of reality began to set in. The initial, simpler path had proven to be a dead end, a hopeful avenue that led only to a brick wall of disappointment. Each negative test was another brick in that wall, and it was growing forbiddingly high. We were at a crossroads, emotionally exhausted and uncertain of which way to turn. It was in this state of weary limbo that our doctor sat us down to have a difficult but necessary conversation. I remember the sterile quiet of his office, the scent of antiseptic cleaner, and the gentle but firm tone of his voice as he explained that while IUI had been a good first step, it was time to consider a more intensive, more aggressive form of treatment: In Vitro Fertilization, or IVF.

The very letters—I-V-F—carried a weight and a stigma that IUI did not. This was the big one, the path that felt less like seeking assistance and more like a full-scale scientific intervention, a surrender to the laboratory. The doctor explained the process, sketching diagrams on a notepad, his pen strokes clinical and precise. It was both fascinating in its scientific intricacy and terrifying in its implications. He described a multi-stage, hormonal marathon. My ovaries would be stimulated with powerful drugs to produce as many eggs as possible, far more than the one or two I would produce in a natural cycle. Those eggs would then be surgically retrieved from my body. In a laboratory, under the watchful eyes of scientists, they would be fertilized with my husband's sperm to create embryos. These tiny, nascent lives, our potential children, would be monitored and graded by embryologists for several days as they grew and divided in a petri dish. Finally, if we were lucky enough—and he stressed the element of chance—to have a healthy, viable embryo, it would be transferred back into my uterus, where we would pray, harder than we had ever prayed before, for it to implant and grow.

It was a path paved with needles, a mountain of hormones, daily pre-dawn appointments, and immense, suffocating financial pressure. But it was also, we were told, our best and perhaps final chance. My husband and I looked at each other across the polished expanse of the doctor's desk, a silent, lightning-fast conversation passing between us. His eyes asked, *Can you do this?* Mine answered, *We have to.* The unspoken question hung heavy in the air: *Are we ready for this?* We had already been through so much. The thought of embarking on an even more demanding, more invasive, and more expensive journey was daunting. But the desire for a child, a desire that had become the central, aching pulse of our lives, was stronger than our fear. With a deep breath that we took in unison and a shared, determined nod, we agreed. We would do whatever it took.

I was not, however, prepared for how completely IVF would take over my life. My kitchen counter, once a place of culinary creation and shared meals, transformed into a mini-pharmacy. It became a sterile, organized collection of vials, syringes, alcohol swabs, and gauze, a clinical landscape in the heart of our home. Every morning began not with a cup of coffee and quiet reflection, but with the nerve-wracking ritual of preparing my injections. I became a reluctant expert in mixing vials of powder and liquid, tapping out air bubbles, drawing precise measurements of medications like Gonal-F and Menopur into a syringe, and finding a new, unbruised spot on my stomach to administer the shot. The small sting of the needle was a minor discomfort, but the emotional weight of it was immense. Every injection was a physical reminder of our struggle, a testament to how far we were from the natural, easy path to parenthood that so many others enjoyed without a second thought.

My body was no longer my own; it was a science project, a vessel being manipulated and monitored with clinical precision. The cocktail of hormones sent me on a wild emotional ride. I would be weepy and fragile one moment, crying over a commercial for pet food, and then filled with an irritable, anxious energy the next, snapping at my husband for no reason. The bloating was a constant, uncomfortable presence, a physical manifestation of the ovarian stimulation that was happening inside me, a painful reminder that my body was being pushed to its limits. I felt disconnected from myself, a passenger in a body being driven by a protocol I didn't fully understand.

The near-daily clinic visits for bloodwork and ultrasounds became a grueling routine. I was still working a demanding full-time job, so my days became a masterclass in logistical planning and emotional suppression. I would have to wake up at the crack of dawn, often before 5 a.m., to drive to the clinic in Rockville, Virginia, or Washington D.C., depending on where we were in the process. I battled the infamous D.C. traffic, my hands clenched on the steering wheel, a silent prayer on my lips that I would make it on time and still get back for a full day of work, where I would have to pretend that my morning had been completely normal.

My husband was my unwavering support through it all. He was there for every single one of those early morning drives, a quiet, steady presence in the passenger seat, his hand a warm anchor on mine. He would hold my hand during the transvaginal ultrasounds, both of us watching the grainy black-and-white screen as the technician measured my follicles. We learned to interpret the images, our hearts leaping with a fragile joy when we saw a multitude of dark, growing circles, a sign that the medications were working. A "good number" of follicles would send a fragile wave of hope through us; a disappointing count would cast a pall over the rest of the day.

From My Husband's Perspective:

Watching Kemi endure the physical demands of IVF was one of the hardest things I have ever had to do. I felt a profound, suffocating sense of helplessness. I could be there, I could drive her, I could hold her hand and pay the ever-mounting bills, but I couldn't take the injections for her. I couldn't endure the physical probing of the ultrasounds. I saw the toll it was taking on her, the way her body was bruised and bloated, the way the hormones affected her moods. She was a warrior, navigating this medical maze with a grace and determination that amazed me. My role was to be her steady rock, her unwavering supporter. But inside, I was a wreck. Every "good-looking follicle" the doctor mentioned sent a jolt of hope through me, a hope so fragile I was terrified to even acknowledge it. I just kept praying silently, asking God to let this be the time, to reward her incredible strength and sacrifice.

Kemi's Perspective:

The most physically demanding part of the process was the egg retrieval. It was a minor surgical procedure, performed under sedation, but it felt monumental. As they wheeled me into the operating room, I would offer up a silent, desperate prayer: *Lord, let there be good eggs. Healthy eggs. Please.* I would wake up from the anesthesia feeling groggy and sore, my abdomen aching as if I'd been punched from the inside out. The recovery was painful, but it was overshadowed by the anxious waiting that followed.

Then came the series of calls from the embryologist, updates that held our entire future in the balance. The first call would tell us the number of eggs retrieved. I remember one cycle where they retrieved nineteen eggs, and we were ecstatic. But then came the brutal attrition of the IVF process. The next call would tell us how many of those eggs were mature. The number would drop. Okay, *fifteen mature. That's still good.* The next day, another call. How many fertilized? The number would drop again. *Ten fertilized.* Then, we would wait day by day as the embryos grew. Day three, how many are still dividing? *Six.* Day five, how many have made it to the blastocyst stage, the stage at which they are viable for transfer? *Two.* It was a brutal, Darwinian Hunger Games, and we were losing potential children at every stage. It was emotionally devastating.

The most emotionally difficult part for me was grappling with the results. To start with so much hope, with nineteen potential chances, and to end up with only one or two, or sometimes none at all, was a unique kind of heartbreak. It was a tangible, numerical representation of our loss.

The embryo transfer itself, however, was a moment of surreal, almost spiritual, hope. We would be in a quiet, softly lit room. On a monitor, we would watch as the embryologist showed us our tiny embryo, a microscopic speck of light that held all of our dreams. We would watch as the doctor carefully threaded a thin catheter into my uterus and, with a gentle push, deposited that speck of light inside me. In that moment, I was what the infertility community calls "PUPO": Pregnant Until Proven Otherwise. For two weeks, I would live in that magical, terrifying limbo, carrying the secret possibility of a new life within me. I would protect my body, eating well, avoiding stress, doing everything in my power to create a welcoming environment for that tiny embryo.

But cycle after cycle, the two-week wait ended with the same crushing phone call. "I'm sorry, Kemi, the test was negative." The hope would vanish, replaced by a grief so profound it felt like a physical illness. It was a constant cycle of hope and despair, a rollercoaster that left us emotionally battered and bruised.

What kept me going? What gave me the strength to endure eleven cycles of this grueling process? It was the word of God. It was my faith, a faith that had been forged and tested in the fires of disappointment. I would ask God for strength for each trip to the clinic, for each injection, for each procedure. I knew, with a certainty that defied my circumstances, that He would see me through. It was a very difficult situation, but my faith was the anchor that kept me from being swept away by the storm.

The physical and emotional challenges of IVF were immense, but they were compounded by the constant pressure from the outside world. The comments from our community, which had started during our early years of marriage, became even more pointed and painful once people knew we were pursuing medical treatment. It was a painful reminder of the cultural double standard that places the burden of infertility so heavily on the woman.

I remember one particularly hurtful encounter when someone laid their hands on my stomach in church, praying loudly for God to heal my "problem." They had no idea of the medical journey I was on, the surgeries I had endured, the daily injections I was taking. Their public display of piety felt like a performance at my expense, reducing my complex and painful struggle to a simple lack of faith that could be fixed with a loud enough prayer. It was humiliating.

Through it all, my husband was there for egg retrievals and transfer of embryos. He was also there for my surgeries, such as fibroid and fallopian tube removal. He was my unwavering support through it all, a quiet, steady presence during the countless early morning drives. He would hold my hand during the trans-vaginal ultrasounds, both of us watching the grainy black-and-white screen as the technician measured my follicles. We learned to interpret the images, our hearts leaping with joy when we saw a multitude of dark, growing circles, a sign that the medications were working. A "good number" of follicles would send a fragile wave of hope through us; a disappointing count would cast a pall over the rest of the day. He was my partner in every sense of the word, sharing the burden of this journey with a strength and a love that never wavered.

I remember another IVF cycle so vividly. That time, I completely changed my lifestyle with the hope of a different outcome. I switched to a plant-based diet, started taking supplements faithfully, and even joined the gym, determined to give my body every possible chance to succeed.

When the cycle began, everything looked so promising. My uterine lining was healthy, my blood work came back strong, and the retrieval went smoothly—we got 9 follicles. Out of those, 6 fertilized, and 3 made it to the blastocyst stage. On day 3, my doctor decided to transfer all 3 embryos, believing that this would increase my chances of finally getting a positive result.

Those two weeks of waiting felt endless. I held on tightly to hope. My body was showing signs, little symptoms that convinced me something was different this time. I thanked God in advance, believing my prayers were finally being answered. I even went out and bought a pregnancy test, my hands shaking as I waited for the result. But when it came back negative, my heart sank.

Still, I clung to Google's reassurance—that sometimes home tests can be wrong. I convinced myself the real confirmation would come from the beta HCG test. On the day of the call, my heart pounded as I waited for the nurse's voice to carry the good news. But instead, I heard the familiar words: *"Kemi, I'm sorry."*

I forced myself to reply, *"It's okay,"* and hung up the phone. The moment the line went dead, so did my composure. I broke down, sobbing uncontrollably, asking myself over and over: *What did I do wrong this time? Why does it always end this way?*

As the years went on, and the number of failed IVF cycles climbed into the double digits, the financial strain became a crushing weight. Our struggle became an open invitation for everyone to offer their opinion, their judgment, or their "miracle cure."

People who had no understanding of the medical complexities would tell me I just needed to "hurry up," as if this was a matter of choice or timing. "Woman's age, it goes quickly," they would say, their words a constant, ticking clock in the back of my mind. "A man can marry at any age and have children," others would add, a cruel insinuation that my husband's future was not as limited as my own. It was a painful reminder of the cultural double standard that places the burden of infertility so heavily on the woman.

The financial sacrifice was immense. We cut back on everything. We gave up vacations, dinners out with friends, new clothes. Every spare dollar was funneled into the "baby fund." It was a constant, grinding pressure that added another layer of stress to our already strained lives.

The final straw came in February of 2020, just before the world shut down with the COVID-19 pandemic. We embarked on our last IVF cycle, our hearts heavy with the weight of so many previous failures. This cycle felt different. The results were the worst we'd ever had. We only retrieved a few eggs. Only one fertilized. Our single, precious embryo. We tracked its progress day by day, our entire future hanging on the fate of a few dividing cells in a petri dish. On day five, we got the call. It wasn't a nurse. It was the doctor herself.

"I'm so sorry, Kemi," she said, her voice heavy with a finality that chilled me to the bone. "The embryo stopped dividing this morning. It arrested."

The word was so clinical, so brutal. *Arrested*. There was no embryo to transfer. There was nothing. Just... silence. The end of the line.

A week later, we sat in her office for a follow-up, the air thick with unspoken grief. She looked at us with deep compassion, her eyes reflecting the years of struggle she had witnessed. "Kemi," she said gently but firmly, "I cannot in good conscience recommend you do another cycle of IVF. Your body has been through enough. We are not getting the results we need."

I looked at her, my mind reeling, not understanding where she was going. And then she said the words that would shatter our world and, eventually, rebuild it.

"If you want to have a biological child," she said, her voice soft but clear, "your best and only remaining option is to use a gestational carrier."

The words hung in the air, a paradox of hope and devastation. A gestational carrier. A surrogate. Another woman would carry our baby. The part of the journey that was mine, a part I had fought for, bled for, and prayed for over a decade—the chance to carry my own child—was being taken from me. My body had failed. It was the final, irrevocable verdict. I started crying, not loud, dramatic sobs, but the quiet, hopeless tears of someone who has nothing left to fight with. The war was over, and I had lost.

This was the breaking point. This was the moment when the path we had been on for fifteen years crumbled into dust. We had endured so much, sacrificed so much, only to arrive at a new, impossibly high wall. The medical journey, as we knew it, was over. We were left with nothing but our broken hearts, our empty bank account, and the daunting, terrifying question of what came next.

Prayer Point:

Lord, thank You for giving us the courage to explore every possibility with wisdom. Guide our decisions and protect

what You have planted. Help us trust You—not just with
the outcome, but with the process. In Jesus' name, Amen.

Chapter 4
THE MEDICAL MAZE

The journey through IVF was not a straight line; it was a labyrinth, a disorienting medical maze of changing clinics, new doctors with different philosophies, and unexpected, often brutal, surgical detours. Looking back, I see a map of our lives marked not by years, but by clinics and cycles. The journey was a relentless pilgrimage from one sterile waiting room to another, a constant search for a new strategy, a different protocol, a flicker of hope that hadn't yet been extinguished. Over the course of more than a decade, we visited five different fertility clinics. Each time we made a change, packing up the heavy binder that held my voluminous medical records—a testament to years of pain—it was born out of a quiet desperation, a feeling that what we were doing wasn't working and that we needed a fresh set of eyes, anything to change the relentless outcome.

Our journey began in Rockville, then moved to a clinic in Virginia, and then to another in the heart of Washington D.C. Each clinic had its own philosophy, its own unique atmosphere of hope and despair. Some were large, bustling centers that felt like factories for baby-making. I remember the cold, impersonal nature of those places. The waiting rooms were packed, the chairs filled with women clutching folders, their faces etched with the same silent anxiety I felt twisting in the pit of my stomach. We were a sisterhood of unspoken sorrow, each of us trying to project an aura of calm while our worlds were crumbling inside. In those places, I was just another number on a chart, a set of hormone levels on a screen. The nurses, though likely doing their best, were always efficient but hurried, their interactions transactional. "Your bloodwork is fine," they'd say without looking up. "The doctor will call you with the next steps." We felt like we were part of a conveyor belt, moving from one station to the next, the process feeling cold, impersonal, and profoundly lonely. I spent hours in those waiting rooms under the low hum of fluorescent lights, trying not to make eye contact with the other women, yet feeling an invisible thread connecting us all. Each of us was there because a fundamental part of our body, a part we were told was our natural purpose, was not working. The shared shame and hope were so thick in the air you could taste it.

Other clinics were smaller, more intimate practices. There, the staff knew my name, and the waiting rooms held only a handful of us at a time. In those quiet spaces, there was a different kind of energy—a shared, unspoken understanding, a quiet solidarity that passed between us with a simple, knowing glance. But in some ways, this intimacy made the inevitable bad news even harder to bear. The phone calls, whether from a brisk, anonymous nurse from the "factory" or a kinder, more familiar one from the smaller practice, always delivered the same devastating blow, a single word—"negative"—that had the power to shatter a month's worth of carefully constructed hope. I learned to brace myself every time the phone rang with the clinic's number, my heart hammering against my ribs, a prayer caught in my throat.

Interspersed between the grueling IVF cycles were a series of surgeries, each one a separate, pitched battle within the larger war we were waging. These weren't minor procedures; they were invasive, painful detours that demanded their own seasons of recovery and grief. I underwent three separate fibroid surgeries. Each time, the process was the same. A doctor would point to shadows on an ultrasound and explain, with clinical precision, how these benign tumors in my uterus might be interfering with implantation. Each time, a fragile hope would ignite within me: *maybe this is it, maybe this is the thing that will finally make it work.* The pre-op anxiety was immense—the fasting, the early morning drive to the hospital, the sterile smell of the operating room. Then came the post-op pain, a deep, internal ache that served as a constant reminder of the battle being fought inside my own body. Each surgery required a significant recovery period, weeks spent in a painful and frustrating pause, my body healing while my spirit grew more weary. It was a brutal cycle: the surgery, the long weeks of recovery, the slow rebuilding of my strength, and then the cautious return to another IVF round, only to be met with the same familiar failure.

When it was time to begin another cycle, I walked into the clinic carrying both fear and faith. The very first step was the baseline ultrasound—the scan that shows if your body is ready to move forward with stimulation medication. I laid on the table, my heart racing, praying for good news.

But as the doctor's eyes lingered on the monitor, I saw her expression change. She turned to me gently and said, *"Kemi, we've found a cyst on your left ovary."*

An ovarian cyst—just a simple, fluid-filled sac—was enough to stop everything. She explained that it could interfere with the growth of healthy follicles, and in some cases even secrete hormones that would disrupt the cycle. The stimulation medications meant to help me could actually make the cyst larger, turning hope into more complications.

So the cycle was canceled before it even began. Just like that, the fragile hope I had been holding on to slipped right through my fingers. I would first need to undergo treatment to remove the cyst before I could try again.

I walked out of the clinic that day feeling like the ground had crumbled beneath me. And now, before I could even take another step forward, I was forced to face yet another setback.

With tears streaming down my face, I whispered to myself, *"Why does this journey have to be so hard? What more does my body have to endure?"*

And yet, in the middle of that crushing moment, there was still a quiet voice inside me—soft but steady—reminding me: *Don't give up.*

Then came the ovarian cyst surgery. After several failed IVF cycles, I was completely shattered. Yet even in my pain, I couldn't let go of hope. I told myself, *"Maybe the next one will be different."* So I picked myself back up, determined to try again.

It felt like a particularly cruel joke from the universe. Just when we thought we had cleared one battlefield, a new enemy appeared on a different front. It was another invasive procedure to address a new problem, another scar on my already weary body. The journey began to feel like a cruel game of whack-a-mole;

every time we summoned the strength and resources to solve one medical issue, another would immediately pop up in its place. My body, which I had once trusted implicitly, now felt like a foreign territory, a landscape of betrayal that I no longer understood. It felt less like a part of me and more like a project I was managing, a series of problems that needed to be solved, none of which had easy answers.

The most devastating of these surgical detours was the one to address an infection in my fallopian tubes. I remember sitting in the doctor's office as she explained, her words clinical and detached, that the infection was severe. The only course of action, she stated, was to remove the tubes entirely. I remember her explaining the medical necessity, but all I could hear was the cold, hard finality in her voice. This surgery would forever close the door on the possibility of a natural pregnancy. While we were already far down the path of IVF, this felt like a point of no return. It was another layer of profound loss, another piece of the natural dream that was being surgically cut away. I remember signing the consent forms, the cheap plastic pen feeling heavy in my hand. The weight of my signature, the black ink on the page, felt like a permanent seal on a future that could never be. The recovery was difficult, not just physically, but emotionally. The new scars on my abdomen were no longer just marks from surgery; they were a permanent, visible reminder of all that had been physically taken from me on this journey. They were a map of my losses.

After years of this grueling cycle, moving from clinic to clinic with no success, I was emotionally and physically exhausted. The constant seesaw of hope and despair had worn me down to a nub. I was on the verge of giving up. And then, just as the darkness felt complete, a dear friend referred me to a new clinic in Bethesda. This clinic, and the doctor I met there, would become a pivotal turning point in our story.

From the moment I met this doctor, I felt a different kind of connection. She was not just a clinician; she was a compassionate partner in my journey. In our first consultation, she did something no other doctor had done: she closed the binder of my medical records, looked me directly in the eye, and asked, "How are *you* doing through all of this?" Tears immediately welled in my eyes. For the first time in a long time, I felt seen not as a collection of failed cycles and problematic test results, but as a human being with a deeply held dream. She took the time to truly listen, to understand the long and painful road I had traveled. Her passion for her work was palpable, and it reignited a spark of hope within me.

I remember her telling me about a free IVF trial the clinic was offering. After reviewing my complex case, she said I qualified. The fact that I was older and had never been pregnant made me a candidate. After years of hemorrhaging our life's savings into this dream, the offer felt like a miracle in itself, an incredible gift and a reprieve from the immense financial pressure we had been under for so long.

We tried the cycle, and unfortunately, it did not result in a pregnancy. The familiar grief washed over me, but for the first time, the failure didn't feel like a final verdict. The doctor's passion and commitment were unwavering. She was not deterred. "Okay," she said, her tone filled with a new resolve. "That didn't work. Now we figure out why."

She delved into my case with a level of detail and curiosity that no other doctor had ever shown. And she was the one who finally noticed something that had been overlooked for years: a lack of sufficient blood circulation in my uterus. This, she believed, was a key factor in our repeated implantation failures. It was a potential answer, a piece of the medical puzzle that had been missing for so long. This doctor was also the one who helped us make a crucial strategic decision. She saw that my body was struggling to produce a high number of quality eggs with each IVF cycle. But we had several frozen embryos from previous cycles, embryos that had been created when I was younger and my egg quality was better. She strongly advised us to preserve these precious frozen embryos. "Continue to use fresh eggs for now," she said with profound wisdom, "but let's keep these embryos safe. They are your best insurance policy for the future." Her advice was a lifeline. She helped us preserve our frozen embryos, a medical decision that would prove to be one of the most important we ever made. She didn't know it then, and neither did we, but she was helping us protect the very children we would one day hold in our arms.

The final wall in the medical maze, the one that truly marked the end of the road, arrived in February of 2020. We embarked on our last IVF cycle with hearts heavy with the weight of so many previous failures. This cycle felt different. The protocol was more aggressive, the injections more potent, and I could feel the immense strain on my body. Every shot was a mixture of hope and dread. My stomach was a canvas of small bruises, a daily testament to the battle. Yet, after years of this war, my body did not respond as we'd hoped. I remember the profound sense of defeat during the ultrasounds, watching the screen and seeing only three follicles develop. Just three. After all that medication, all that effort, that was it. Of those, only one fertilized. Our entire medical journey, every surgery and every scar, now rested on a single, precious embryo. We tracked its progress for five agonizing days, our entire future hanging on the fate of a few dividing cells in a petri dish. Every morning I woke up with a knot in my stomach, wondering, *Is it still dividing? Is it still growing?*

Then came the call that ended the medical war. I saw the clinic's number on my phone and my breath caught in my chest. It wasn't a nurse. It was the doctor herself. Her voice was gentle, but her words were clinical steel. "I'm so sorry, Kemi," she said. "The embryo stopped dividing this morning. It arrested." The world went quiet around me. All I could hear was that one word, echoing in the silence. *Arrested.* A word for a criminal, not for a nascent life. A word that was so brutal, so cold, so final.

A week later, we sat in her office, the air thick with unspoken grief. She looked at us with a compassion that came from witnessing years of our struggle. "Kemi," she said, her voice both kind and firm, "I cannot in good conscience recommend you do another cycle of IVF. Your body has been through enough. We have to stop." There was no other option offered, no new strategy to try. The maze had come to a dead end. Medically, the journey was over, and we were left with nothing but the quiet, sterile finality of her words and the daunting, terrifying question of what could possibly come next.

Prayer Point:

Heavenly Father, thank You for turning our waiting into dancing. Thank You for Tobi and Tomi—living proof that You are faithful. May their lives reflect Your glory. May every couple still waiting receive strength and assurance that You are never late. In Jesus name. Amen!

Chapter 5
CULTURAL PRESSURES AND FAITH STRUGGLES

The journey through infertility is not just a medical battle; it is a profound spiritual and emotional war, fought on multiple fronts. The daily injections, the invasive procedures, the clinical disappointments—those were battles fought within the quiet confines of a hospital. But for me, the most challenging front, the one that waged war on my spirit every single day, was the constant, grinding pressure of my own culture. Coming from Nigeria, where having children immediately after marriage is not just a preference but a deeply ingrained expectation, my childlessness was a public spectacle. It was an unspoken headline attached to my name, a source of endless commentary, unsolicited advice, and sorrowful, pitying glances that felt like tiny paper cuts on my soul. My every move, my every interaction, was viewed through the lens of my empty womb. It was a heavy, suffocating weight to carry, an invisible cloak of failure that I could never take off, especially at family gatherings and community events where the joy of others' children only magnified my own perceived lack.

The year 2012 was a particularly brutal one. In March, my world was shattered by the sudden loss of my mother. She was my rock, my biggest cheerleader, the one who had been with me every step of the way on this fertility journey. She was more than just a supportive parent; she was an active partner in my fight. I remember her sitting at her dining table for hours, poring over medical journals and newspaper clippings, her brow furrowed in concentration. She would research IVF clinics for me, cutting out articles about new treatments and sending them to me with hopeful, handwritten notes in the margins. Her faith was practical and fierce. She was the one who, with unwavering conviction, would take my hands, look me in the eye, and say, "Kemi, don't worry. I know you are going to have children." Her belief in my dream was a powerful source of strength for me, a shield against the doubts that constantly tried to creep in. Her sudden passing left a gaping hole in my heart, a void that felt both personal and strategic. I had lost not just my mother, but my greatest spiritual ally in this war. My family—my father, my siblings, and I—were all reeling from the shock and the grief.

It was in this raw, vulnerable state, just two months later in May, that I experienced one of the most bizarre and painful encounters of my life. We were at a friend's husband's 50th birthday party. The atmosphere was celebratory, filled with the sounds of laughter and highlife music, but my heart was still heavy with mourning. I felt like I was moving through the world behind a pane of glass, present but not truly connected. I was trying my best to smile, to engage in small talk, when a woman I barely knew, a guest of another guest, approached me. She had a certain look in her eye, a predatory curiosity that immediately set my nerves on edge. She looked me up and down, a slow, deliberate appraisal that made me feel like an insect under a microscope. Her gaze was filled with a strange, unsettling mixture of pity and accusation.

"How come you haven't gotten pregnant?" she asked, her voice loud enough for those around us to hear. The question, so direct and invasive, hung in the air, silencing the chatter around me. "What's going on?"

I was stunned into silence. My mind went blank. What could I possibly say? Should I detail my years of failed treatments, my surgeries, my grief, right here on the dance floor? Before I could even formulate a response, she leaned in closer, her inquiry taking a dark, spiritual turn. "When you sleep, do you see children?" she pressed, her voice dropping to a conspiratorial whisper that felt more like a hiss. "Are you an *ogbanje*?"

The word hit me like a physical blow. In our culture, an *ogbanje* is not just a mischievous spirit; it is a spirit child, an evil entity believed to be part of a demonic fraternity, one who torments a family by being born and dying repeatedly, delighting in the cyclical pain of its parents. To be asked if I was one was not just an insult; it was a spiritual accusation of the highest order. It was a suggestion that my infertility was not a medical issue, but a manifestation of evil. It implied that I, myself, was the source of my own barrenness, that my spirit was tainted, that I was demonic.

I was shocked, confused, and deeply hurt. I was still grieving the loss of my mother, the very woman who had been my spiritual shield, and now I was being accused of being in league with demons. The cruelty of it, the sheer insensitivity of attacking someone in their most vulnerable moment of grief, was breathtaking. I couldn't hold back the tears. They welled up and spilled over, hot and shameful, as I stood there, exposed and assaulted, in the middle of a party. My fresh grief, so raw and close to the surface, was now compounded by this strange and painful spiritual attack. This encounter was a stark example of the kind of pressure I was under. It wasn't just about having a baby; it was about my spiritual standing, my very identity as a woman of faith.

Mother's Day became another annual source of pain. The day was already difficult because of my longing for a child, a dull ache that sharpened with every smiling family photo I saw on social media, with every sermon dedicated to the joys of motherhood. But after my mother's death, it became a day of double grief. I mourned the mother I had lost and the mother I had not yet become. The emptiness felt cavernous. And every year, my pain was compounded by the careless words of one particular woman. In our culture, it is common to wish all women, regardless of their maternal status, a "Happy Mother's Day" as a sign of respect for their nurturing spirit. It's a gesture of communal acknowledgment. But this woman, every single year, would make a point of finding me and, with a saccharine smile, saying, "Oh, when you become a mother, I will wish you a happy Mother's Day."

Her words shocked me every time. They were a deliberate, calculated exclusion. Why would a grown woman say something so deliberately cruel? Does having children biologically make you a mother? Are women who adopt not mothers? Are women who nurture and mentor not mothers? Her narrow, judgmental definition of motherhood was a denial of my worth, a public declaration that, in her eyes, I was incomplete. In our culture, you can't talk back to someone who is older than you; you are expected to be silent and respectful. So I would just nod, my anger and hurt churning inside me, feeling silenced and shamed.

It was not a pleasant experience. I would go home and ask God, "Why? Why would someone say that to me?" It felt like a spiritual assault, weaponizing a day of honor to inflict pain.

The spiritual pressure came from all sides. People would tell me I should go to a church in South Africa to see a famous prophet. Others would suggest I call a pastor who could go to the mountains to pray for me. It was amazing how many people had a "solution" for my problem, how many people assumed my infertility was a spiritual issue that required a special intervention. I would look at them, these people who should know better, and be amazed at their presumption. Their advice, though perhaps well-intentioned, carried an implicit judgment: that my own faith, my own church, my own prayers, were insufficient. They were subtly telling me I wasn't doing enough, wasn't holy enough, wasn't connected enough to God to solve my own problem.

I thank God for the Word that was instilled in me, the faith that anchored me through these storms. I did not believe what these people said. I chose to believe what the Word of God said. I stood on His promises. In the quiet of my room, I would say to myself, "God, you have promised that I will be called Mother. I will be a mother." And I held on to that word, to that promise, with everything I had, even when my circumstances screamed the opposite.

It was in the midst of this challenging environment that my community of true supporters became my lifeline. I thank God for my friends. I thank God for my community. They were the ones who were supportive during this whole process. My friend Abiodun, whom I call Abbey, and I would have prayer meetings every week. She created a safe space where I didn't have to be strong. I could just let it all out—the anger, the frustration, the grief—and she would just listen, never judging. And then she would pray for me, her faith a shield when my own was riddled with holes, encouraging me and reminding me of God's faithfulness. Her friendship was a gift of immeasurable worth.

I also had a circle of supportive friends like Ebere and Ram. My high school friend in Nigeria, Bunmi, was a relentless source of hope, always sending me lists of clinics to check out, always encouraging me to not give up. She was the one who first mentioned surrogacy to me, planting a seed long before I was ready to even consider it. My friend Abbey also mentioned it, but at the time, I wasn't interested. It wasn't something that was done in our community. I didn't know anyone around me who had done it. It wasn't until Ram told me about her co-worker that the idea began to take root.

I had spent years building a fortress of faith to protect myself from these attacks, standing on God's promises when the world offered only judgment. I held fast to the belief that my story would prove them wrong, that God's faithfulness would be my vindication.

When I finally started to consider this new, foreign path, I reached out to my pastor, Chrys. She didn't hesitate. "Oh yeah," she said, her voice filled with encouragement. "Why don't you give it a try?" Her simple, faith-filled endorsement was a powerful confirmation. I also had lunch with another friend, Idong, at Panera Bread, and she pushed me and encouraged me to explore the option. I had lots of friends who were very supportive during this period, who, in spite of all the cultural pressures, used the word of God to encourage me. I thank God for my supporters. It's just so good to be surrounded with people that will uphold you, people that will hold you accountable, people that will pray for you when you can't pray for yourself. When you don't have the strength to pray, you need people like that in your life.

Then, in 2020, the clinical verdict landed. Our last IVF embryo arrested, and the doctor confirmed my body could not carry a child.

For me, this was more than a medical failure; it felt like a spiritual one. The cruel whispers of the woman who questioned my spirit at the party, the painful jabs on Mother's Day declaring I was not yet complete—they all came rushing back, no longer as whispers, but as a deafening roar of validation for my deepest fears. It felt as though every judgmental voice had been proven right. In the darkness of my room, my prayers were no longer pleas; they were accusations. 'God, why?' I cried out, the words torn from a place of profound betrayal. 'After all this, was my faith not enough? After all my trust in You, were *they* right about me all along? Have you forgotten me?'

The doctor's words had ended the medical battle, but they had ignited a much deeper crisis. It was the most painful test of my life. The war for my faith itself was hanging in the balance, and I was terrified of which side would win.

Prayer Point:

Lord, in the midst of the battle, when the pits of despair feel overwhelming, be our strength. When our faith is tested and our hearts are broken, remind us that You are our fortress. Give us the courage to stand on Your promises, even when the world's judgment is loud and our circumstances feel hopeless. In Jesus' name, Amen.

Chapter 6
The Breaking Point

The year 2020 was a breaking point, not just for the world, but for me. After fifteen years of relentless, hope-fueled striving, I came to the end of my road. The final IVF cycle we attempted, right before the COVID-19 pandemic shut everything down, was different from all the others. The medications were more aggressive, but my body, weary from years of hormonal manipulation and surgical interventions, did not respond well. I was only able to produce three eggs. Of those three, only one fertilized. Our entire, multi-decade hope was pinned on that single, microscopic embryo.

We watched it for five agonizing days, our prayers a constant, desperate whisper. And then came the call from our doctor, her voice heavy with a finality that chilled me to the bone. "I'm so sorry, Kemi," she said. "The embryo stopped dividing this morning. It arrested."

That was it. That was the break. The moment when the last ember of hope seemed to be extinguished. In a follow-up conversation, our doctor told us, with a kindness that was both gentle and firm, that she would not recommend any more IVF cycles. "Kemi," she said, "your body has been through enough. We have to stop." Then she uttered the words that would both shatter our world and, eventually, rebuild it: "You will have to use a gestational carrier."

I realized then that this was serious. This was the final word. The path of trying to carry my own child was over. So, I did what I had always done: I reached out to my community. I told my family the devastating news. I told my circle of friends. I told my pastor. People offered their condolences, their prayers, their recommendations. And I began my own research. I retained a lawyer to help me understand the legal complexities of surrogacy. She recommended different sites for me to check out, and I began to delve into the world of gestational carriers.

I spoke with a woman who used a surrogate, and she generously shared her experience with me. But as I learned more, a new, insurmountable wall began to rise before me: the cost! In the United States, the price of a surrogacy journey was over $200,000. It was an impossible sum, a staggering, heartbreaking figure that felt like a cruel joke. After all we had been through, after all we had sacrificed, were we now going to be priced out of our miracle?

In a moment of desperation, I reached out to my brother, who works at a bank, and to my sister. "Do any banks offer 0% interest rate loans for something like this?" I asked, my voice trembling with the humility of having to ask. Their response, though likely well-intentioned, was another painful blow. "No, Kemi," they said. "You shouldn't even go that route. Why do you want to get into debt for this? You should just trust God. He will do it for you."

I was so disappointed, so hurt. I thought, Wow. They don't understand. We had been trusting God for nearly two decades. We believed this new path was where He was leading us. To be told to just keep waiting, to just "trust God" without taking any action, felt like a profound misunderstanding of our agonizing journey.

It was in this place of absolute brokenness that I knew I needed help. I had to deal with the trauma of all that I had been through. I started therapy, a decision that was life-changing. In 2020, in the midst of the global uncertainty of the COVID-19 pandemic, I began to unpack the accumulated grief of the last fifteen years. It was a loss, a huge loss, and I had to mourn it properly. My therapist helped me through this process. She helped me realize that my inability to carry a pregnancy did not make me less of a woman, less of a mother. It was an amazing journey of healing and self-discovery, of dealing with the rejections and the trauma I had endured for so long.

It was also a time of intense practical preparation. We knew that this new path, if we chose to take it, would be expensive. We started saving aggressively, cutting down on so many expenses. It was a mental and financial preparation for a journey we weren't even sure was possible. We had to cut down on a lot of things we used to do. It was another sacrifice, another step of faith into the unknown.

It was during this time that a new, unexpected idea began to surface. My friend, Abiodun, had mentioned surrogacy in Nigeria to me before, but I hadn't listened. I wasn't ready. Then, my friend Ram told me about a co-worker of hers who had gone through the process in Nigeria. I was intrigued. Is this really possible? I wondered. To ship an embryo from the USA to another continent, to a different environment? They assured me that it was, that there were companies that specialized in exactly that.

Even with this new possibility, I knew I had to convince my husband. He was not on board at first.

From My Husband's Perspective:

When Kemi first brought up the idea of using a gestational carrier, I was resistant. It was not what we had signed up for. It felt foreign, strange, and risky. But I knew I had to pray about it. As I prayed, I began to see it differently. I thought about the concept of adoption, of loving a child that was not biologically yours. And then I thought, Well, these are our biological children. They are our embryos. We are just using a different method to bring them into the world.

Kemi's Perspective:

I used another analogy to help him see it from a different perspective. "Mary was a gestational carrier for God," I said. "The seed was from the Holy Spirit, not from Joseph. God Himself used this method to bring Jesus into the world." I wasn't comparing our situation to the birth of Christ, of course, but I wanted to show him that God can work in unconventional ways. We sometimes bash science, but science has helped so many people. We talk about kidney transplants, heart transplants—these are all miracles of science. We shouldn't ignore the gift of science. I thank God for it.

This new perspective began to soften his heart. He started to see the possibility, the hope, in this new, unexpected path. He began to appreciate the miracle of it all, the way an embryo, a tiny collection of cells, could develop into a fully formed human being. He started to get excited.

I am so grateful to have seen the whole process of the development of my children. That's something I can never forget, seeing them going from cells to developing into embryos, changing in shape and size over time in the pictures, seeing the ultrasound, everything. It's something that forever will stay in my heart. I will be forever grateful. It's so it's an amazing journey, even though it was painful, but at the end of the day, it was worth it, it was worth it to see my beautiful children. It was worth it to see that consistency does pay off.

In our Yoruba culture, names are not just labels; they are prophecies, declarations of destiny, and reflections of a family's journey. We named our daughter Oluwatomilola, which means "God's blessings are sufficient for me." We call her Tomi. This name is a daily reminder to me that my worth, my sufficiency, is not found in myself, but in Him. For all the years I felt inadequate, less than, a failure as a woman, this name is a declaration of truth: His grace is enough. Our son is named Oluwatobiloba, which means "God is a big God," or more literally, "God is a great king." We call him Tobi. This name is a testament to the fact that our God is bigger than our problems, bigger than our pain, bigger than our doubt. He is a great king who reigns over all circumstances.

Their English names, too, are imbued with meaning. Our son is Joshua, named for the biblical leader who, after years of wandering in the wilderness, brought his people into the Promised Land. Our daughter is Hannah, named for the woman in the Bible who endured the pain of barrenness and the taunts of her rival, but who never gave up praying for a child. Her name also means "grace" or "favor," a constant reminder that our children are a gift of God's unmerited favor.

When they are old enough, we will tell them the stories behind their names. We will tell them, as it says in Psalm 78:4, "the praiseworthy deeds of the Lord." Their very names will be a testimony to His faithfulness.

The timing of their birth also held a deep, personal significance for me. Our twins were born on November 3rd, the day after my mother's birthday. My mom, who had been my greatest cheerleader, my tireless researcher, my unwavering source of faith, never got to meet her grandchildren. Her passing in 2012 left a void in my life that I thought would never be filled. Mother's Day, which had always been a painful reminder of my own childlessness, became a day of double grief after she was gone. But God, in His infinite wisdom and kindness, wove her memory into the fabric of our joy. Now, her birthday and our children's birthdays will forever be linked. Mother's Day, which used to be a painful reminder of grief, has become bittersweet. It's a time when I honor my mother's legacy by celebrating my own miraculous path to motherhood. I know she was rejoicing in heaven when Tomi and Tobi were born.

The story of Jacob's wife, Rachel, in the book of Genesis, has also taken on a new meaning for me. After years of infertility, when she finally held her son, Joseph, in her arms, she cried out, "God has taken away my disgrace." I understand that feeling so deeply. For years, I wrestled with the shame of my infertility, a shame that was compounded by the judgments and assumptions of others. But like Rachel, my story did not end there. She named her son Joseph, which means "may he add," a declaration of faith that the God who had given her one child could give her more. Rachel knew she served a God who multiplies his blessings.

Her sister, Leah, also chose meaningful names for her children. She was unloved by her husband, and God saw her distress. She named her first son Reuben, which sounds similar to the Hebrew for "He has seen my misery." Her next son was Simeon, meaning "one who hears," and her last was named Judah, meaning "praise." Leah and Rachel chose names that reflected the providence of God and His active role in their journeys to motherhood.

Names are important to God. In the Bible, He has many of his own: Jehovah-Jireh, "The Lord will provide"; Jehovah-Rapha, "The Lord that Heals"; El Shaddai, "Lord God Almighty." The name Jesus itself translates to "God saves." What we call ourselves matters, and what we call our children matters. It is the first prayer we speak over their lives.

The arrival of our twins was not without its own set of challenges. Their due date was November 23rd, but they decided to make their grand entrance on November 3rd, at just 35 weeks. We had already bought our tickets to arrive in Nigeria on November 15th. I received the call at work that the gestational carrier was having continuous contractions and that they would have to perform a C-section. Our lives changed in an instant. I had to change my ticket and pay an extra $600 that we hadn't planned for.

The sonogram had shown two girls, so we were completely shocked when we discovered on the day of delivery that we had a boy and a girl. We had picked out names for two girls, but thankfully, the Nigerian names we had chosen were unisex. We just had to find a new English name for our son that very day, so it could be on the birth certificate. That's how he became Joshua.

We never met the surrogate. The process was anonymous, and while a part of me was curious, I am also grateful for the simplicity of it. She was a vessel, a blessing, an answer to our prayers, and I will be forever grateful for her selfless act. But our connection was to our children, and that was all that mattered.

Holding them for the first time was the most profound, emotional moment of my life. All the pain, all the waiting, all the tears—everything was worth it for this. It was a long, eleven-hour flight home, and the journey was challenging with two tiny infants. But they handled it beautifully. And when we finally walked through our own front door, a family of four, the silence of our home was finally, blessedly broken. The journey was over, and we were home.

Prayer Point:

Lord, when we are at our breaking point, when our hope is exhausted and the path behind us is filled with pain, meet us in our brokenness. From the ashes of our disap-

pointment, show us the new path You are creating. Grant us the courage to take the first step into the unknown, trusting that You are already there, and the grace to heal from the battles behind us. Amen.

Chapter 7
THE COMMUNITY THAT CARRIED US

The journey through infertility can be an incredibly isolating one. It's a private war waged behind a public smile, a grief that is often invisible to the outside world. For years, my husband and I felt like we were adrift on a vast, lonely ocean, fighting the waves by ourselves. It was a strange and lonely existence, marked by a painful duality. Publicly, we were a happy, successful couple, active in our careers and in our church. We celebrated with friends at their baby showers, held their newborns, and offered our sincere congratulations, all while a silent scream echoed in our own hearts. Privately, our lives were a landscape of clinical procedures, hormonal injections, and a grief so constant it had become a part of our very breathing. As we look back now, we can see that even in the loneliest stretches of that ocean, God had placed lighthouses all along our path—friends, family, and a community of believers who refused to let us drown. They were the ones who held up our arms when we were too weak to fight, who loaned us their faith when ours was depleted, and who ultimately became the hands and feet of the miracle we were praying for.

This wasn't always the case. In the early years, the voices of judgment and misunderstanding, as I've shared, were often the loudest. But even then, there were glimmers of true, Christ-like support that sustained us, small pockets of grace that reminded us we were not entirely alone.

One of the earliest and most poignant examples of this happened in 2006. We were only a few years into our medical journey, still reeling from the initial shock of failed treatments. Our hope was fragile, and our pain was raw. A few of my dear friends—Vivian, among them—decided they were not going to let us walk this path alone. They came together and threw me a baby shower.

I was shocked, stunned into disbelief, when they told me. A baby shower? For a woman who wasn't pregnant and had no prospects of becoming pregnant anytime soon? The idea seemed absurd, almost cruel. My first instinct was to say no. A party felt like a public spectacle of my failure, an invitation for more pitying glances and whispered condolences. I was terrified of sitting in a room full of women, opening gifts for a child that existed only in my dreams, the potential for humiliation and heartbreak felt immense. But they insisted. It was not a shower to celebrate a baby, they explained; it was a shower to celebrate a promise. It was an act of audacious faith, a prophetic declaration that the baby we were praying for was already on its way.

Reluctantly, I agreed. I remember walking into that room, my heart braced for impact, but what I found was not a room of pity, but a sanctuary of hope. It was filled with women who had come not to mourn with me, but to prophesy over me. They didn't bring gifts for a hypothetical baby; they brought gifts of encouragement, of Scripture, of prayers written on beautiful cards that I still have to this day. It was an incredibly moving and healing experience. The most astonishing moment came when my friend Vivian handed me her gift. I unwrapped it to find two small outfits: one for a boy and one for a girl. "For the twins," she said with a confident, knowing smile. I laughed, a sound of pure, overwhelmed disbelief. Twins weren't even on my radar; I was just desperately praying for one healthy child. But Vivian was planting a seed of faith for something bigger than I could imagine, a prophecy that would take seventeen years to come to pass. That day, I felt seen and loved, not for the mother I might one day become, but for the woman I was, right there in the midst of my struggle. It felt like people do care. You know, there are people that do care, and I thank God for them.

This was the community that began to form our shield. It included pillars of faith like Mommy Fawole, a woman whose steadfast belief and gentle encouragement were a constant comfort. She wasn't a typical Nigerian mother, bound by the cultural expectations that so often caused me pain. Her focus was not on the timeline of tradition, but on the timelessness of God's promises. Her faith was not loud or demanding; it was a quiet, unshakeable confidence in God's goodness that she poured into me every time we spoke. She would call just to say she was praying, her voice a calm anchor in my turbulent emotions. She treated me not as a woman who was lacking, but as a daughter who was waiting on a loving Father. Her belief was a powerful antidote to the judgmental voices that surrounded me.

Our Bishop and his wife, Pastor Chrys, were also significant anchors in our community. From the pulpit and in private, they modeled a faith that was not just hopeful, but certain. They were always praying for us and, more importantly, thanking God in advance for the children they *knew* we would have. They never wavered. Their sermons would often speak of God's faithfulness in the waiting, and I always felt they were speaking directly to me, strengthening my resolve. Their leadership created an atmosphere within our church family where faith for our future was the norm. Our church became a place where our dream was nurtured, not questioned. The collective belief of our church family was a powerful force, a spiritual incubator for the miracle that was to come.

My friend Abiodun, whom I call Abbey, was my prayer partner and my rock through the darkest parts of the medical journey. She was with me through every single IVF cycle. She was there from beginning to the end. She was supportive, praying for me through my chemical losses, she was there, very supportive. So I really think I really thank God for her. She was the one I would call from the car, my voice choked with tears after another negative result, unable to even form the words. She wouldn't offer easy platitudes or simple solutions; she would just listen, creating a sacred space in the silence for my grief. And then she would pray, her faith a shield when my own was full of holes.

And there was Mama C, another pillar of faith in my life. She would call me every Monday without fail, just to pray with me. Her consistency was a lifeline in a journey marked by the devastating inconsistency of my own body. She didn't just pray from a distance; she visited me in the hospital during one of my surgeries, bringing her faith and comfort right to my bedside when I needed it most.

From My Husband's Perspective:

Having a community that supported Kemi was everything. While I was her primary support, I knew there were places in her heart that only another woman, another friend, could reach. Watching these women rally around her was an answer to my own silent prayers. They understood her pain in a way I couldn't, and their friendship was a balm to her soul. It also strengthened me, knowing she wasn't alone when I was at work or when I simply didn't have the right words. Our community held both of us.

Kemi's Perspective:

The most powerful and humbling demonstration of this support came after we hit rock bottom in 2020. The door to IVF had been slammed shut, and the path to surrogacy seemed financially impossible. We were heartbroken, defeated, and had no idea what to do next. We had shared our devastating news with our closest circle of friends and our pastor. We weren't asking for anything; we were just sharing our pain.

A few weeks later, we received a call. A small group from our community—our friends, our prayer partners—had been meeting in secret. They had heard our story. They had seen our pain. And they had decided, as a body of believers, to act. "We want to help," they said. "We are going to help you raise the money for the surrogacy."

I was floored. I didn't know how to react. Accepting help on that scale was incredibly difficult. My pride bristled at the thought of being a charity case. It's one thing to accept a casserole or a card; it's another thing entirely to accept thousands of dollars from the people you worship with every Sunday. But my therapist had been preparing me for this. She had taught me about the grace of receiving, about allowing others the blessing of giving. She reminded me that being vulnerable and allowing the community to step in was an act of faith in itself.

And so, with humility and overwhelming gratitude, we said yes.

What followed was one of the most miraculous displays of God's provision we have ever witnessed. Word of our need spread quietly among the friends, family, and church members we had confided in. There was no formal fundraising, no public campaign; it was a sacred, personal movement of the heart. People felt moved to give, and they did so with incredible generosity and love. They gave sacrificially, not out of pity, but out of a shared belief in the promise we were standing on. We received checks and transfers, some from people we knew well, others from members of our church family we barely knew, all with notes that said, "We are praying for you and believing with you." It was the church in its purest form, a living embodiment of James 2:15-16: "Suppose a brother or a sister is without clothes and daily food. If one of you says to them, 'Go in peace; keep warm and well fed,' but does nothing about their physical needs, what good is it?" Our community didn't just offer us prayers; they provided the financial miracle that made the next step possible.

This outpouring of support taught us a profound lesson. We had spent so many years feeling like we were on the outside looking in, a childless couple in a family-focused world. But in our moment of greatest need, our community wrapped its arms around us and pulled us into the very center of its heart. They showed us that we were not a problem to be solved, but a part of the body to be loved and supported.

This journey also gave us the opportunity to support others. We had advised a couple struggling with infertility to pursue a gestational carrier, sharing what we had learned. When they followed that path and welcomed a child, their joy became our joy. It was a beautiful reminder that even in our own waiting, our story could be a source of hope and guidance for others. God was using our pain for a purpose far beyond ourselves.

Therapy taught me about self-care, and community taught me about corporate care. It taught me that it's not only okay to need help; it's essential. We were not created to bear our burdens alone. The weight of our infertility journey was too heavy for two people to carry. But when it was distributed among a community of faith, it became bearable. They didn't just carry the financial load; they carried the emotional load, the spiritual load. They were the tangible, walking, talking, giving evidence of God's faithfulness. They were the body of Christ, and they carried us to our miracle.

The support we received from our community was not just emotional and spiritual; it was intensely practical. When we finally made the decision to pursue surrogacy in Nigeria, our friends were the ones who helped us navigate the overwhelming logistics. They were the ones who said the right thing at the right time, encouraging us and reminding us to trust God through the daunting process of international coordination and shipping our precious embryos across an ocean. They held us accountable. Even when I was scared of taking the risk, they were there, making sure that I was following through, asking, "Kemi, when are you doing this? What's the next step?" I really thank God for them. My community means so much to me, and I want to thank God for them.

This journey has taught me the vital importance of being plugged into a community. I encourage everyone to find their people, to be intentional about building a support system. But it's not just about receiving support; it's also about giving it. We have to be there for one another. We can't just expect things to come our way; we have to be givers as well. During that period, my friends were so very, very supportive, and their example has inspired me to be just as supportive to others in their time of need.

Therapy was another crucial form of support that helped me prepare for the new life that was coming. My life was good, but it was about to change in a way I couldn't even imagine. Therapy helped me to get ready for that change, to appreciate who I am in Christ, even when I was doubting myself. Sometimes, you just need someone to say the right thing to you, to reflect the truth of who you are back to you when you can't see it for yourself. I was doubting myself, but I thank God that He made it possible to have people around me that would push me and help me to bring out the best version of myself. I thank God for them.

The years we spent waiting for children were agonizing, but I can now see that they were also a blessing in disguise. God gave us the time we needed to prepare to be the best parents possible. The years we spent working provided us with the financial security we needed to start a family. I also sought therapy to work through my own childhood hurts and the emotional toll of infertility. I wanted to be a rock for my children, a source of encouragement and strength, and God used all of those years to refine me for His purposes. None of them were wasted. Seeking therapy, working on our finances, avoiding negativity, and leaning on our supportive community were all crucial in navigating this journey.

Our testimony is a beacon of hope for couples facing similar struggles, encouraging them to trust in God's faithfulness and never give up on their dreams of parenthood. The community that carried us was a living, breathing example of God's love in action. They were the hands that held us up, the voices that prayed for us, the hearts that believed with us. We could not have done it without them. And for that, we will be eternally grateful.

Prayer Point:

Heavenly Father, we thank you for the incredible gift of community. Thank you for the friends, family, and believers who stand with us, who pray for us, and who become Your hands and feet when we are too weak to stand on our own. Help us to not only graciously receive this support but to also become a source of that same strength and encouragement for others on their journey. Remind us that we are never truly alone. In Jesus' name, Amen.

Chapter 8
A New Path Opens

The weeks following the doctor's final verdict were a desolate landscape of grief. We had hit rock bottom. The fifteen-year road of intensive medical intervention in the United States had ended not with a gentle exit, but by falling off a cliff. The door to me carrying my own child was permanently closed, and the only alternative suggested—a gestational carrier in the U.S.—was locked behind a financial wall so high it seemed insurmountable. We were emotionally, physically, and financially bankrupt. The dream, for all intents and purposes, felt dead.

We existed in a heavy fog. Days bled into one another, marked by a quiet, shared sorrow. The silence in our home was different now. It was no longer the silence of anxious waiting, but the hollow echo of defeat. We had no plan, no next step, no direction. All we had was the rubble of our broken hearts and a faith that was being tested in the deepest fire it had ever known.

It was in this place of absolute emptiness that God chose to plant a seed, not with a thunderous voice from heaven, but in a casual conversation after a community event. I was at the African Heritage Festival, an event I loved, surrounded by the vibrant sounds and sights of my culture. My friend Ram approached me, her expression gentle but purposeful. She told me she had been speaking with our mutual friend, Ebere, who had been at that faith-filled baby shower in 2006 and had witnessed our long journey.

"Kemi," Ram said, her tone purposeful. "I've been meaning to tell you something. A co-worker of mine... she and her husband had been struggling for years, just like you. They ended up using a surrogate in Nigeria."

I stared at her, my mind struggling to process her words. Nigeria? The idea was so far outside the realm of what I had ever considered that it sounded like something from a movie. My immediate thoughts were a cascade of fear and skepticism. *How is that even possible? Is it safe? Can their medical standards be trusted? How could you manage something so sensitive and complex from thousands of miles away?* I had heard of international adoption, but international surrogacy felt like a completely different universe. I had always thought that surrogacy was something only rich people could afford, and the idea of attempting it across an ocean seemed not just reckless, but impossible.

I was amazed that such a thing existed, but I thanked her for the information, and we exchanged a few voice notes with her co-worker, asking questions and getting a sense of her experience. But inside, I initially dismissed it as an unworkable, high-risk fantasy. We had just been crushed by the logistical and financial impossibility of surrogacy in our own country; the thought of attempting it across an ocean seemed ludicrous.

I brought the idea home to my husband, expecting him to dismiss it as quickly as I had.

From My Husband's Perspective:

I was still reeling from the concept of surrogacy at all. The idea of another woman carrying our child was a massive emotional and theological hurdle I was struggling to clear. When Kemi mentioned "surrogacy in Nigeria," every alarm bell in my system went off. It felt like taking an already terrifying idea and multiplying the risk by a thousand. "Absolutely not," I said, more firmly than I'd intended. "It's out of the question. We don't know anything about it. It's too far, too risky. We have to draw a line somewhere." My resistance wasn't just about logistics; it was about self-preservation. I had watched my wife endure years of physical and emotional trauma. The thought of embarking on a new, unknown venture that could lead to even more heartbreak was something I couldn't bear. I wanted to protect her, to protect us, from more pain. The door, in my mind, was closed.

Kemi's Perspective:

But the seed Ram had planted in my mind, though initially dismissed, had taken root. In the days that followed, I couldn't shake the conversation. Despite my husband's firm no, and despite my own fears, a tiny, persistent voice in my spirit kept whispering, "What if?" Fueled by a desperation that overrode my skepticism, I started digging. I did my research. I discovered that the clinic Ram's friend had used was a highly reputable one in Nigeria. Then, a second confirmation came. My high school friend in Nigeria, Bunmi, had also mentioned this very same clinic to me in the past. The pieces began to connect.

I decided I was going to give it a try. I was going to push forward. I was amazed at the possibility and I decided to pursue it. I did my research, spoke to the doctor at the Nigerian clinic via a virtual consultation, and they confirmed that the process was straightforward. I contacted my clinic in D.C., and they began to coordinate the paperwork. Everything was set in motion.

My husband, however, was still silent. Not in a bad way, but in a way that I recognized as fear. He had seen me hurt so many times, had witnessed so many disappointments, that he was scared to hope again. He was worried about this new, unknown path. He wasn't as engaged in the process as I was, and I understood why. The weight of our past failures was heavy on him. He was being protective of my heart, and of his own. But I knew I had to keep moving forward.

My conviction grew stronger with each new piece of information. The clinic in Lagos was highly recommended, not just by my friend's co-worker and my friend Bunmi, but by several others I connected with. This clinic stood out. I also did research on other clinics, even in the Caribbean, but I kept coming back to this one. The sheer number of positive testimonials and referrals gave me a sense of peace and confirmation.

I remember discussing my fears with my therapist. I was worried about the distance, about managing such a sensitive process from so far away. We prayed together, and she encouraged me to follow the leading of the Holy Spirit. She also reminded me of a powerful truth: "God wants godly seeds to fill the earth." Her words motivated me, reminding me that this was not just a personal desire, but a spiritual mission.

As a practical step, and a step of faith, I paid $3,500 to retain a lawyer who specialized in adoption and surrogacy law in the United States. This was my backup plan. In the hopes that if the surrogacy in Nigeria didn't work out, I could proceed with adoption. The lawyer was there to guide me, to help me understand the laws, to ensure that whatever path we took, we were protected.

With all these pieces in place—the research, the referrals, the legal counsel, the spiritual confirmation—I was ready. My husband, seeing my determination and the clear hand of God in the details, finally came on board. His fear gave way to a cautious faith, and we became a team once again, ready to take this new, improbable, and exciting step together.

Our nineteen-year journey was not just a quest for a child; it was a profound and often painful classroom where we learned invaluable lessons about marriage, about faith, and about the very nature of God Himself. When my husband and I got married, we never could have anticipated the challenges that would arise, the years we would spend waiting to become parents. This journey was anything but easy, yet it ultimately strengthened our marriage in ways we never could have imagined. All those nights spent praying and crying together brought us closer to God and to one another. We discovered more about ourselves and God's purpose for our lives than we ever would have in a life of ease.

Kemi's Perspective:

Over the years, I remained committed to finding a way for us to have children. I took off work for Kemi's surgeries and drove her to countless appointments. It was hard for me to watch her suffer through all of those procedures, but I never stopped encouraging her or gave up on our dream. Scripture talks about marriage as becoming one flesh, and it was our collective faith that sustained us through trial after trial. We learned to embody biblical love, the patient love that bears all things, believes all things, hopes all things, and endures all things.

At times, we faced challenges that felt insurmountable. One complication led to another as our chances of having children became increasingly slim. But no matter the giants in our way, God was always bigger. Humans can be narrow-minded and think there's only one way forward. When traditional paths to conception failed, it was tempting to think that we'd never have children. "Maybe we should just give up and move on with our lives," the enemy whispered. But we knew that nothing is impossible for God. He sees a million possibilities we never even would have considered. God is faithful to fulfill His promises, no matter how hopeless our circumstances may seem. He is light in the darkness, the one who makes a way in the wilderness and streams in the wasteland. We can trust Him with everything we have because He gave up everything for us, not even sparing His own Son. He withholds no good thing from us. So when we walk through the valley of the shadow of death, we don't have to be afraid. Even if we sink to the depths, God is there with us. He was with us on every step of this journey as a faithful Father and friend.

Our journey to parenthood was not without opposition. We fought spiritual battles against a real enemy who sought to kill, steal, and destroy our faith. At times, the enemy used other people to tear us down. It was especially disheartening when other Christians blamed us for our struggles with infertility. And yet, the challenges that people judged us for were the very circumstances that displayed the power of God in our lives. In our weakness, He became our strength and sufficiency. He stepped into our pain when others ran away. Jesus isn't afraid to get his hands dirty; he went to the places no one else would go to heal the sick, the broken, and the lost. So while our vulnerabilities weren't always met with compassion from others, they demonstrated our need for a savior. They led us to the feet of Jesus—right where we were meant to be.

Even when people criticized me, God never left my side. His plan always prevails, no matter how the enemy tries to detract from His glory. Jesus already defeated death on the cross, so it's a losing fight for the devil. No one can interfere with the purposes of our God, the author and creator of the universe. Love always wins in the end.

At times, this battle became too much for us to fight on our own. I enlisted the help of a Christian therapist, who encouraged me to hold onto my faith even when all hope seemed lost. My therapist taught me the importance of rest and self-care. After every setback, I needed time to recuperate and remind myself of the faithfulness of God. Taking care of my mental and spiritual health was critical to sustaining the endurance it took to keep fighting for our family.

Coming to terms with surrogacy was a journey in itself, a process of surrendering control in a way I never had before. While the research and referrals brought a sense of practical peace, my heart was still a battleground of fear and hope. I remember one specific conversation with my therapist where I confessed my deepest fear: "What if I can't connect with a baby that I don't carry?" It was a raw, vulnerable moment. She encouraged me to see the surrogate not as a replacement for me, but as a helper, an answered prayer, an angel God was sending to help us complete our family. That conversation was a turning point, helping me reframe the journey from one of loss to one of divinely orchestrated help.

Once my husband and I were united in our decision, the process moved forward with a clear timeline. The entire journey, from our first official 'yes' to the day of the embryo transfer, took approximately seven months. The first three months were dedicated to legal arrangements, coordinating between our U.S. clinic and the one in Lagos, and the complex logistics of shipping our frozen embryos. One of the most nerve-wracking events was waiting for the email confirming their safe arrival. For 48 hours, I barely slept, imagining a thousand things that could go wrong. The relief I felt when we received the confirmation was immense; it was the first sign that we were on the right path.

The next step was the selection of the surrogate. Who chose the surrogate? The clinic handled it entirely. We put our trust in their medical and ethical standards. They explained their rigorous screening process: they only worked with healthy women, typically in their late 20s or early 30s, who had already had at least one successful pregnancy and were financially stable. They conducted thorough medical and psychological evaluations to ensure the candidate was fully prepared for the emotional and physical commitment. As for the decision about being anonymous, that was the clinic's standard policy. They explained it was for the emotional protection of both the carrier and the intended parents. While a part of me was curious, we agreed that anonymity was the healthiest path for everyone involved. In March, they informed us they had found a wonderful candidate who met all the criteria. The final months were spent medically syncing her cycle with the hormonal protocol needed to prepare her uterus for the transfer. It was a period of intense prayer and hope, a tangible step toward the miracle we had waited so long for.

Infertility treatments and complications put a strain on our finances. We sought biblical wisdom on how to manage our expenses, trusting God to provide. He did this by pointing us down the path to a gestational carrier and providing support through trusted friends and family. The Lord promises blessings for those who persevere through trials (James 1:12). In fact, in Isaiah 61:7 he says that "instead of shame you will have a double portion." Indeed, God gave us the double blessing of twins.

The birth of our children made the enormous financial and emotional cost of this journey worthwhile. All those years of waiting also gave us time to get our finances in order so that we were prepared to support our growing family. Finances were yet another domain we learned to surrender to God, trusting him to provide for us as we pursued his will.

"We walk by faith and not by sight," Paul writes in 2 Corinthians 5:7. There were many times in this journey when all we could see were roadblocks, but we chose to walk by faith. What if David had been intimidated by Goliath's stature and put his slingshot down? Or if Noah had ignored God's warnings and never built the ark? Faith is what keeps us in step with the will of God. He is strong enough to take down our giants; all we have to do is believe.

We trusted God even when the odds were stacked against us, knowing there is more to life than what we can see. Every physical reality is rooted in a spiritual battle. Jesus has already defeated death, so we can walk in victory even through the most trying circumstances. The Lord knows exactly where he's leading us. All we have to do is follow.

Our journey taught us patience, resilience, and unwavering faith, reminding us of Isaiah 40:31: "But those who trust in the Lord will find new strength. They will soar high on wings like eagles. They will run and not grow weary. They will walk and not faint." Our story is a testament to the power of faith and the unwavering love of God. No matter the challenges, God's plan is always perfect. Trust in Him, and He will provide. We hope that our journey will inspire and uplift those walking a similar path, reminding them that they are never alone and that faith can indeed move mountains.

Prayer Point:

Father, thank You for opening doors we never could have imagined and for planting seeds of hope in the most unexpected ways. When a new and unconventional path appears before us, grant us the wisdom to see Your hand in it. Align our hearts as husband and wife, so we may walk forward in unity. Replace our fear with faith, and our skepticism with a spirit of hopeful trust in Your guidance. Amen.

Chapter 9

SHIPPING HOPE ACROSS AN OCEAN

With the decision finally made to pursue surrogacy in Nigeria, a fragile but persistent hope began to bloom in the barren landscape of our hearts. Yet, as soon as we took one step forward in faith, we were immediately confronted with our next surreal challenge: how, exactly, do you get precious, microscopic embryos from a freezer in a clinic in the U.S. all the way to Lagos, Nigeria? The very concept felt like something plucked from the pages of a science fiction novel.

This challenge was actually the second phase of a journey our embryos had already begun. For years, our embryos rested quietly in a freezer in Rockville, Maryland—little vessels of promise, carrying the hopes and prayers of our hearts. When God led us to switch clinics, they first had to be moved to our new clinic in Washington, D.C. But before that could happen, there was a mountain in our way: an unpaid storage fee from over three years.

When I saw the total, my heart sank. It felt impossible, another financial wall designed to keep us from moving forward. But God already had the provision in place. Out of nowhere, I received a bonus from work—more than enough to clear the debt. That was no coincidence; that was God making a way.

With the fees paid, we faced the next hurdle. Hiring a special medical transport to move the embryos from Rockville to D.C. would have cost over $1,000—money we didn't have. So, the task of carrying this precious cargo fell to us. The Rockville clinic gave us strict instructions: the embryos had to be kept absolutely secure, avoid all bumps, and arrive in D.C. in under 45 minutes.

We prepared the car like it was holy ground. My husband moved the passenger seat forward so the precious container could be pressed snugly against the back seat, with no room for movement. We planned the drive for after rush hour, and I remember telling my husband, "Please, no speeding—steady, careful, prayerful."

That drive felt like a sacred mission. My hands were clenched, my heart was praying without ceasing. Each bump avoided, each turn taken gently, was covered in a silent prayer: *Lord, protect them... Lord, bring us there safely.* It wasn't just a trip from Rockville to D.C. It was faith in motion. It was hope in the back seat. And it was yet another reminder that the God who begins a good work is faithful to carry it through.

Now, with our embryos safely in Washington D.C., we faced the even more daunting task of sending them across an ocean. This was not a package we could simply insure and send via FedEx. These were our future children, our only biological link to the family we had dreamed of for two decades. Our entire legacy, every hope and prayer, would be placed into a specialized, state-of-the-art metal canister and sent on a journey across continents in the cargo hold of an airplane. The thought was both terrifying and utterly humbling.

The moment the decision was made, I wrapped the entire endeavor in a thick blanket of prayer. I knew we could not navigate this alone. I immediately informed my prayer warriors—my steadfast friend Abbey, my insightful friends Ram and Ebere, and our beloved pastor, Chrys. They became our spiritual ground crew, keeping us in the loop of their prayers, interceding constantly for the safe passage of our precious cargo. I also confided in my other close friends, including my facial consultant, LaRay. During one of my appointments, as she worked, I shared the latest, improbable turn in our story. A fellow believer, her eyes lit up with encouragement. "Kemi," she said with a certainty that bolstered my own wavering faith, "you will be a mother." After that first facial, our relationship deepened into a friendship, and her words became another confirmation that God was surrounding me with faith-filled people for this next, unbelievable leg of the journey. The support was a tangible force, a wave of hope and prayer lifting us up.

The process, which had seemed so daunting at first, began to unfold with a smoothness that could only be described as divinely orchestrated. Our clinic in Washington D.C., and our new clinic in Lagos began to coordinate everything. The logistical hub of the whole operation was a specialized medical logistics company called Cryoport. They are the experts in shipping precious frozen embryos, sperm, and eggs around the world in high-tech metal canisters, called dewars, which are filled with liquid nitrogen to keep their precious cargo at a stable, sub-zero temperature. The six-hour time difference between Maryland and Nigeria wasn't a major issue for me; after years of juggling a demanding career, I was used to coordinating across time zones. My primary, all-consuming concern was the safe arrival of our embryos.

The day the embryos were scheduled to be picked up from our D.C. clinic was a day of immense surrender. We had done everything we could. Now, it was out of our hands. We had to trust God, and we had to trust the process. We paid the substantial fee to Cryoport, and they took care of the rest.

But of course, while the logistics were straightforward, the emotional journey was anything but. We tracked the shipment online, every update a tiny heartbeat of reassurance. We watched as our embryos, our tiny, frozen hopes, traveled from Washington D.C. to a layover in Europe, and then finally, to Lagos. The act of shipping my embryos, my faith, my future, across the ocean was an immense leap of faith. I was so scared. I wasn't sure what the outcome would be, and the weight of it all was immense. And then, after days of holding our breath, we received the email we had been praying for: the embryos had arrived safely. Everything was fine. A wave of relief so powerful it almost brought me to my knees washed over me. The first, and perhaps most improbable, leg of our journey was complete.

But with the embryos landed in Lagos, a new wave of anxiety took its place. They first had to be carefully thawed and tested for viability by the clinic's embryologist to ensure they had survived the journey. Would they survive the journey? Would the change in environment, the transfer from one lab to another, affect them? The questions were relentless.

With the embryos safely in Lagos, the next phase began: the selection of our surrogate. This was another step that required a huge amount of faith and trust, especially after the years of trauma that had led me to this point. I was so grateful for my community during this time. My friends and pastor were praying for us, and God also sent encouragement from the most unexpected places.

The clinic in Nigeria was incredibly helpful and transparent. My doctor and my nurse were my primary points of contact, and they guided me through the whole process. Our consultations were virtual, and my doctor was so kind and reassuring that it put my anxieties at ease.

They explained their rigorous screening process for surrogates. They were looking for a woman who was young, healthy, and had already had at least one child of her own. In March, they found a candidate who met all the requirements. She passed all the medical and psychological screenings, and we were kept in the loop every step of the way. We had to sign legal paperwork, of course, but the clinic handled everything with a secure professionalism and a smoothness that was truly a blessing.

I was nervous, of course. I would text my doctor every now and then with questions, and she was always so patient with me. She understood what I was dealing with—the anxiety, the fear, the years of trauma that had led me to this point. She would tell me that my feelings were normal, and her team made me feel sure that this was a viable, safe, and professional path.

The therapy I had been doing also played a crucial role in preparing me for this stage of the journey. I had learned to process the loss of not being able to carry a pregnancy myself, and that healing was crucial in allowing me to embrace this new path with an open heart. So, while this process was filled with anxiety about the unknown, it wasn't as bad as it could have been, because I was emotionally prepared. I was ready to trust God with the outcome. When God opens a door, He makes a way.

Once the surrogate was selected and all the legal paperwork was signed, the medical process began in earnest. The clinic synced our surrogate's cycle with a hormonal protocol to prepare her uterus for the embryo transfer. We received regular updates, tracking her progress from afar. It was a strange and surreal experience to be so intimately involved in, yet so physically detached from, a medical procedure affecting another woman's body for our sake.

From My Husband's Perspective:

I was still processing the idea of surrogacy, and to be honest, I was not as engaged in the day-to-day details as Kemi was. It wasn't that I wasn't supportive, but I was scared. I had seen her hurt so many times, had witnessed so many disappointments, that a part of me was still guarded, still fearful of another heartbreak. I could understand why she was so determined to push forward, but for me, the years of disappointment had taken their toll. I was worried about this new path, this new opportunity for hope to be crushed. My silence during this time was not a lack of interest; it was a shield, a way of protecting my own heart from more pain.

Finally, the day of the embryo transfer arrived. We knew the exact time it was scheduled to happen in Lagos. Back in Maryland, we stopped everything. We spent that hour in fervent prayer. We pictured the embryologist carefully selecting our two best embryos. We pictured the doctor performing the transfer. We pictured our two microscopic hopes, our tiny specks of light, being placed into the safe, welcoming space of her womb. We prayed for the skill of the doctors, for the health of our surrogate, and for the embryos to implant and grow. We released them, with both trembling hands and faithful hearts, into the care of God.

And then, once again, we entered the torment of the two-week wait.

This time, however, it was different. We were not obsessively analyzing every twinge in our own bodies. The wait was quieter, less physically consuming, but no less intense. The fate of our future was completely out of our hands, unfolding in a place we could not see. It was the ultimate exercise in trust. Every day, we would pray together, casting our anxieties on God and standing on His promises.

The day the pregnancy test was scheduled was April 1, 2023. We were acutely aware of the date—April Fool's Day. We prayed it wouldn't be a cruel cosmic joke. The time difference meant we would likely get the news in the early morning, our time.

Prayer Point:

Lord, we entrust what is most precious to us into Your hands. As we send our hopes across the miles, be the guardian of this journey. Grant us peace when the outcome is out of our hands, and quiet our anxious hearts. We thank you for the helpers and the prayer warriors You place around us, our spiritual ground crew. May Your favor go before us in every detail. Amen.

Chapter 10
The Call That Changed Everything

The call—or rather, the text—that changed everything came on a day the world reserves for jokes and pranks. It was April 1, 2023. April Fool's Day. A day for harmless deception and laughter. But for us, it would become a day of profound, unbelievable blessing, a day when God's truth felt more real and miraculous than any fiction.

I woke up that Saturday morning to the familiar rhythm of a weekend. The air in our home was buzzing with the ordinary energy of a day off. I believe it was around 7:38 a.m. when my husband and I were getting ready to go to the gym, with a quick stop at Sam's Club planned for our usual weekend shopping. It was a day like any other, which made the miracle that was about to unfold feel all the more stunning. As I was in the car, my phone buzzed with a text message. It was from our doctor in Nigeria. My heart leaped into my throat, a frantic, hopeful drumbeat against my ribs. My hands were shaking so much I could barely hold the phone steady. I took a deep breath and read the four words that would unravel nineteen years of pain:

"Congratulations, your GC is pregnant."

The world stopped. Pregnant. The word I had longed to see, to hear, to feel for two decades was finally, unequivocally, ours. I let out a sound that was half sob, half shout. My husband, who was in the driver's seat, looked over at me, his face a mask of concern. I couldn't speak. I just held out the phone for him to see. He read the text, his eyes widening in disbelief. "Wow," he whispered, his voice thick with emotion. "Is this real?"

It was so surreal, so momentous, that our minds couldn't immediately accept it. We just sat there in the car, stuck for a moment, the world moving around us while we were suspended in a bubble of shock and overwhelming joy. I started to cry, not the quiet, sorrowful tears of grief I knew so well, but a flood of joyous, cleansing, cathartic tears. All the years of pain, of disappointment, of silent cries and monthly goodbyes—it all came pouring out, washed away by a single, beautiful word.

We drove to Sam's Club, our original plan feeling laughably mundane in the face of this life-altering news. We were in a daze. I remember walking into the cavernous warehouse store, the bright lights and bustling shoppers feeling like a different reality. We were supposed to be buying groceries, but we just wandered the aisles, aimlessly pushing an empty cart, looking at each other every few minutes and bursting into laughter. We couldn't concentrate. We couldn't shop. It was quite amazing. We left the store without buying a single thing, got back in the car, and headed to the gym, still in a state of shock. But we couldn't even exercise. We just left the gym, our hearts and minds buzzing with an energy that had nothing to do with a physical workout. We were just amazed.

That evening, we began to share our news. I called my friends. I called my family. I told our pastor, Chrys. Each conversation was a fresh explosion of thanksgiving and praise. "She's pregnant!" I would say, the words feeling more real each time I spoke them. Everyone was just rejoicing with us. It was April 1st, and while some might call it April Fool's Day, for us, it was April Blessing's Day. It was the day God's promise began to take shape in the most tangible way imaginable. I will always remember April 1st.

The initial confirmation, however, was just the beginning. The clinic needed to monitor the pregnancy hormone (hCG) levels every two days to ensure they were doubling as they should—a sign of a healthy, progressing pregnancy. This brought a new kind of anxious waiting. But with each test, the news was good. The numbers were strong. They were multiplying beautifully.

Then came the first ultrasound, scheduled for April 11th. We waited anxiously for the report. The call came, and the news was another shockwave.

"Everything looks great," the nurse said cheerfully. "And we saw not one, but two heartbeats."

Twins. The prophecy from my friend Vivian at that baby shower seventeen years earlier came rushing back to me. I just laughed, a sound of pure, giddy disbelief. Two? After all this time, after praying for just one, God was giving us two? It was overwhelming, terrifying, and absolutely wonderful all at once. I thought, "Okay, God, what is going on?" One child is a challenge, but we were going to have to double everything—double the diapers, double the feedings, double the love. It was a beautiful, chaotic, and perfect fulfillment of a promise we had almost given up on.

We were just thanking God. But our journey has taught us that the path to a miracle is rarely a straight one. A few weeks later, we faced another terrifying ordeal. After a routine ultrasound, we received a report from a different doctor at the clinic. The report confirmed the healthy, growing heartbeat of one baby, but then came the devastating sentence: they couldn't find the second embryo. The sac, they said, appeared to be empty.

I began to worry. The old, familiar fear, which had been dormant for a few blissful weeks, came rushing back in, cold and suffocating. I immediately told my friends what the doctor had said. "Oh God," I cried, "how can this be so? What happened?" They told me they didn't know, that the sac just seemed to have stopped growing. It was a devastating blow. To be given the joy of two, only to have one snatched away, felt like a cruelty beyond measure.

The next day, I had a previously scheduled session with my therapist. I told her the news, my voice choked with grief. She listened patiently, and then she looked at me with a gentle but firm intensity. "Kemi," she said, her voice a challenge, "whose report will you believe?"

Her question cut through the fog of my grief like a bolt of lightning. The doctor's report was one of fear, of what could be seen with human eyes. But there was another report, a higher report.

"I will believe God's report," I said, my voice shaky but resolute.

"Good," she replied. "And what does the Bible say?"

She reminded me of God's promise: "No one shall die, but we shall live to declare the works of God." She encouraged me to continue to proclaim that word, to believe that with long life, the Lord would satisfy me and my children.

Her words ignited a fire in my spirit. I went home from that session a different woman. I was no longer a passive victim of circumstances; I was a warrior heading into battle. I opened my Bible, and another scripture resonated deep in my heart, Romans 8:11: "But if the Spirit of Him who raised Jesus from the dead dwells in you, He who raised Christ from the dead will also give life to your mortal bodies through His Spirit who dwells in you."

I began to meditate on that scripture, to claim it, to pray it over my children. I personalized it, my voice growing stronger with each repetition: "If the Spirit of Him who raised Jesus from the dead dwells in me, He who raised Christ from the dead will also give life to my babies' mortal bodies!" I was claiming the promises of God, speaking life over a situation that looked like death.

For two long weeks, I lived in that space of active, defiant faith. I refused to mourn the child the doctor's report had declared lost. Instead, I prayed with a new intensity, a new focus. I was not just hoping; I was warring in the spirit, standing on the authority of God's word. I told my friends, my prayer warriors, to stand with me, to believe God's report, not the doctor's.

The following week, our regular doctor performed another ultrasound. The first one, the one with the bad report, had been done by a different doctor at the clinic. This time, our trusted physician was at the helm. After the scan, she sent me a video clip. My husband and I huddled together, our hearts in our throats, as we pressed play. The screen was filled with the familiar black-and-white image of the ultrasound.

And then we saw it. A strong, steady, rhythmic flicker. One heartbeat.

And right next to it, another. Just as strong, just as steady. A second heartbeat.

"We found the true heartbeat," our doctor's voice narrated over the video, filled with a gentle joy. "Both are strong."

Man, that was just God. The relief that washed over us was so powerful it felt like a physical wave. We just erupted in praise, thanking God for His faithfulness, for His goodness. I had been so worried, and in a moment, He had turned our fear into a profound sense of awe. We were glorifying God for how He had made everything possible. To God be the glory. We give Him all the honor for what He has done, because it is truly Him that made this possible. It was a scare, but God turned everything around for our good. What the enemy meant for evil, God turned it around. And today, we have our joy, we have our miracles. Thank you, Jesus.

This experience taught me a powerful lesson about faith. It's not about denying reality; it's about choosing to believe in a higher reality. It's about knowing that God's report is the final one, and that His power is not limited by what we can see or understand.

The rest of the pregnancy progressed smoothly. Every two weeks, we would receive our ultrasound updates, and with each report, our hearts would swell with gratitude. The babies were growing, their heart rates were strong, and everything was going well. We thank God for the life of our gestational carrier, our helper. She was doing well, and we were so happy that she was able to be a blessing to us.

This journey, from the initial shock of the pregnancy news to the terrifying scare and the ultimate victory, was a microcosm of our entire nineteen-year walk. It was a journey of breathtaking highs and devastating lows, of fear and faith, of human frailty and divine intervention. It was a testament to the fact that even when the path is fraught with challenges, God is always in control. He is a God who can turn a bad report into a good one, who can bring life out of what seems like an empty situation, and who can make a way where there seems to be no way. The call that changed everything on April 1st was not just a text message from a doctor; it was a declaration from heaven that our season of weeping was over, and our season of joy had begun.

I had plans to attend an event called *Emerge*. I was scheduled to be there, smiling, welcoming guests as they arrived. But of course, everything changed after the call.

Prayer Point:

Lord, we thank You that Your report is the final report. When we are faced with news that brings fear and doubt, help us to stand on Your promises. Give us the faith to believe what we cannot see and to trust that You can turn any bad report into a testimony of Your glory. Remind us that Your power is not limited by human circumstances. In Jesus' name, Amen.

Chapter 11
Preparing for Miracles

After the terrifying ultrasound scare and the subsequent, faith-affirming confirmation that both of our babies were healthy, we settled into a new phase of the journey: preparing for a miracle. The pregnancy progressed smoothly. Every two weeks, we would receive our ultrasound updates from the clinic in Lagos. With each report, each new image of our growing children, the reality of our situation became more tangible. Their heart rates were strong, their growth was on track, and everything was going well. We were so grateful for our gestational carrier, our helper, who was providing a safe and nurturing environment for our babies to grow. We were happy that she was able to be a blessing to us, and we prayed for her health and well-being every day.

We knew from the beginning that a twin pregnancy was considered high-risk, and that the babies would likely arrive early. Their official due date was November 23rd, but our doctors had prepared us for a delivery around 35 or 36 weeks. With that in mind, we booked our flights to travel to Nigeria on November 15th, giving us what we thought was a comfortable buffer.

A strange thing happened during this time. For some reason, I felt a strong, persistent nudge from the Holy Spirit to start preparing for our trip, long before it seemed necessary. Months before our scheduled departure, I started buying things, packing suitcases. My husband thought I was crazy. "Why are you doing this so early?" he'd ask, laughing at me. "We have plenty of time." But I couldn't explain it. I just felt a clear prompting to start doing this now. So, I packed the babies' clothes, their blankets, their bottles—everything they would need. I packed my own hospital bag. Everything was ready, everything was literally packed. The only thing I hadn't packed were my own clothes, but all the baby stuff was ready to go. I didn't know why I was doing it, but I obeyed the prompting.

The call that changed everything came on Friday, November 3rd. It was a day after my late mother's birthday, a day that was always tinged with a bit of sadness and remembrance for me. I was at work, sitting at my desk, when my phone rang. It was the clinic in Lagos.

"Kemi," the case manager said, her voice calm but firm. "The surrogate is having continuous contractions. We are taking her to the hospital. The babies are coming today. You need to prepare for your emergency travel."

I froze, the phone pressed to my ear. Today? But our tickets were for November 15th. That was twelve days away. Panic began to bubble up inside me. I immediately called my husband, my voice trembling. "They're coming. They're coming now."

What followed was a flurry of frantic activity. I had to call the airline and pay a hefty fee—$600 that we hadn't budgeted for—to change my flight to leave that very night. I called my boss, my COO, my coworkers, explaining the situation. They were all incredibly supportive, telling me to go and not worry about a thing. My friends swooped in to help. One friend's husband, a tech expert, rushed over to my house to help me pack up my work computer. I was in a daze, my mind racing, trying to process the sudden, dramatic shift in our timeline.

The clinic called again. It was 10 p.m. in Nigeria, around 6 p.m. our time. They told me that they would have to perform a C-section. The babies had to come out because the doctors were concerned about their heart rates dropping. "Wow," I thought, my heart pounding. They said they would keep us posted. Then they asked me a question that brought the reality of our situation into sharp focus: "Who do you know in Nigeria that can get to the hospital to help?"

My sister-in-law, Buki, immediately came to mind. She and her family lived in Lagos. I called her, my voice shaking as I explained the situation. She dropped everything. I think of her life, her own responsibilities, her own family, and yet, in that moment of crisis, she dropped everything and raced to the hospital. She was caught off guard, but she didn't hesitate. She became our feet on the ground, our family representative, our angel in a moment of beautiful, chaotic crisis. She was the one who was there to help buy the first things our babies would need, to help with the first feedings of milk. I will forever thank God for her life, for her selfless love and support.

As I sat on the plane that night, flying across the Atlantic alone, a whirlwind of emotions swirled within me. There was fear for the health of our babies, born so early at only 35 weeks. There was anxiety about the logistics awaiting me in Nigeria. But overriding it all was an overwhelming sense of awe. I thought of the suitcases, already packed and waiting by the door. I thought of my mother's birthday, just the day before. It felt as if God and my mother were orchestrating this from heaven, a bittersweet and beautiful welcome for her grandchildren.

I was just praying for their well-being, for them to be healthy and strong. My sister-in-law was sending me videos and pictures from the hospital. The nurses and the doctors were also sending me updates. I was seeing my children for the first time on a tiny phone screen, thousands of miles away. It was then, staring at those first precious images, that I learned the final, beautiful surprise of our journey. The clinic had told us that it looked like we were having two girls, but they had put a question mark on the report, unsure of the gender of the second baby. A wise friend had advised me to buy neutral colors, just in case, and I had listened. Now, I understood why. The C-section had gone smoothly. Our babies were here. They were healthy. And from the pictures, it was clear: they were not two girls.

It was a boy and a girl.

A boy and a girl. The news was a shock, a delightful, joyful surprise that sent another wave of wonder through my already overwhelmed heart. We had picked out names for two girls. We had prepared our minds and our hearts for two daughters. And now, in a moment, everything had changed again. I remembered my friend's advice to buy neutral-colored clothes, and I thanked God for her wisdom. Our Nigerian names, thankfully, were unisex, but we had to come up with a new English name for our son, right there on the spot, so it could be put on his birth certificate. And so, in a moment of inspired joy, he became Joshua. It was a perfect, unexpected twist in our already incredible story.

When I finally landed in Lagos, I was exhausted but running on pure adrenaline. Buki picked me up, and we went straight to the hospital. I remember walking into that hospital room, my heart pounding. I hadn't packed any clothes for myself, just for the babies. I was about to meet my children for the first time. The thought was both exhilarating and terrifying.

The first time I held them is a moment that is etched in my memory forever. The nurse gently lifted my son, Tobi, and placed him in my arms. He was so tiny, so fragile, weighing just five pounds. I looked down at his perfect face, his delicate eyelashes resting on his cheeks, his tiny fingers curled into a fist. And I began to cry. It wasn't the wracking sob of grief I had known for so long; it was a deep, cleansing release, the sound of a nineteen-year drought ending in a flood of pure, grateful joy.

Then, they placed my daughter, Tomi, in my arms. At just four pounds, she felt as light as a feather, a precious, beautiful miracle. As I held them, one in each arm, the weight of their small bodies was nothing compared to the immense weight that was lifted from my heart. I just stared at them, examining every feature, trying to memorize them. Does he look like me? Does she have her father's nose? They were real. They were human beings. They were my children. I could not believe it. It was a beautiful, overwhelming, and profoundly humbling experience.

When we found out we had a boy, I was so confused that I had to ask my sister-in-law, "Are they sure? Are you sure that's a boy?" She just laughed and said, "Yes, Kemi, look at the picture!" I was so shocked. But the shock soon gave way to a new layer of joy. My husband is the only son of his parents, and the cultural pressure to have a son to carry on the family name had been another unspoken weight on our journey. I knew he had held a private hope for a son. And now, God, in His extravagant grace, had given him his heart's desire.

The hospital in Lagos was a blur of motion and sound, but for me, time stood still. I had just flown across an ocean on a wave of pure adrenaline, my mind a chaotic whirlwind of fear and frantic prayer. Now, standing at the threshold of the neonatal unit, a profound and holy quiet settled over my spirit. A nurse, her face wreathed in a kind smile that spoke of shared joys she had witnessed a thousand times, led me toward two small, transparent bassinets. And there they were. My children. Tobi and Tomi. For nineteen years, they had been a faceless, nameless dream, a persistent, aching hope. Now, they were real. They were breathing. They had tiny, perfect fingernails. They were mine.

From My Husband's Perspective:

When Kemi sent me the pictures from the hospital in Nigeria—the ones the clinic and Buki had sent before she even traveled—and I realized we had a son, I was ecstatic. I was dancing with joy. A son! After all these years, after all the waiting, God had given us a son. It was a moment of pure, unadulterated happiness. I couldn't wait to get to Nigeria, to hold him, to hold both of my children. The feeling was indescribable. I was no longer just a husband; I was a father. A daddy.

As for the surrogate, we never met her. The process was completely anonymous, which, in the end, was a blessing. It allowed us to focus all of our emotional energy on our children, on the new family that was being born. She was an instrument of God's grace, a vessel for our miracle, and we will be forever grateful for her selfless act. But our journey was with our children, and that was where our focus needed to be.

Kemi's Perspective:

I had arrived in Nigeria with nothing but the clothes on my back and suitcases full of baby things. I had to go out and buy clothes and other necessities for myself, a surreal and joyful errand. For two weeks, I was there on my own with the babies, waiting for my husband to arrive on his originally scheduled flight. It was an exhausting and beautiful time of bonding, of learning the rhythms of my new life as a mother of two.

When my husband finally arrived and held his children for the first time, it was a moment of profound, holy significance. The look on his face, a mixture of awe, joy, and overwhelming love, was something I will never forget. Our family was finally complete, all of us together in the same room for the first time.

All the pain, all the waiting, all the years of questions—it all melted away in that moment. Tobi and Tomi had made their grand entrance into the world, strong, healthy, and more beautiful than we could have ever imagined. The names we had whispered in prayers, the faces we had seen only in our dreams, were now real. They had faces, hands, eyes, and voices. Our long-awaited song had finally begun.

Prayer Point:

Heavenly Father, we stand in awe of Your extravagant mercy and abundant blessings. You are a God of beautiful surprises, the one who orchestrates details we could never imagine. We praise You for Your perfect timing and Your tender care. Thank You for not only meeting our needs but for delighting our hearts with unexpected joy. May we never forget the wonder of Your goodness. Amen.

Chapter 12
The Arrival of Joy

I approached their bedsides, my legs unsteady as if walking on water. The nurse gently lifted my son, Tobi, and placed him in my arms. He was so tiny, so fragile, yet so solid and warm. He weighed just five pounds, but he felt like the weight of the entire world, a precious, grounding presence. I looked down at his perfect face, his delicate eyelashes resting on his cheeks, his tiny fingers, with their miniature nails, curled into a fist. And I began to cry. It wasn't the wracking sob of grief I had known for so long; it was a deep, cleansing release, the sound of a nineteen-year drought ending in a flood of pure, grateful joy. All the years of pain, the invasive questions, the medical procedures, the crushing disappointments—every single tear I had ever shed for this moment felt like it was being redeemed. He was here. He was real. I was no longer just a wife, a sister, a daughter. I was a mother.

Next, they placed my daughter, Tomi, in my arms. At just four pounds, she felt as light as a feather, a precious, beautiful miracle who had fought to be here. As I held them, one in each arm, the weight of their small bodies was nothing compared to the immense weight that was lifted from my heart. The constant, grinding burden of childlessness, a weight I had carried for so long I had forgotten what it felt like to be without it, was gone. In its place was a love so fierce and overwhelming it left me breathless. I just stared at them, examining every feature, trying to memorize them. *Does he look like me? Does she have her father's nose?* It was a surreal and beautiful inventory of a dream made flesh.

I was alone in that moment, but not lonely. My husband was still in the U.S., preparing to join me. My friends and family were celebrating from afar. But in that quiet hospital room, surrounded by the beeps and hums of medical equipment, I felt a profound sense of victory. I had held onto faith in the darkness, and God had brought me into the glorious light.

The first few days were a surreal blend of exhaustion and exhilaration. I stayed by their side, learning the rhythms of their tiny lives—the sleepy yawns, the hungry cries, the peaceful sighs. My sister-in-law, Buki, was my angel on earth. She had dropped everything to be there, and she helped me navigate the overwhelming first days. She helped us buy milk, diapers, and all the things I hadn't had time to prepare for a boy and a girl. Her presence was a tangible expression of the family support that had been a cornerstone of our journey.

From My Husband's Perspective:

The two weeks I had to wait in Maryland before flying to Nigeria were the longest of my life. I was a father, but my children were on the other side of the world. Kemi would send me a constant stream of pictures and videos. I would stare at my phone for hours, memorizing their faces, marveling at every tiny detail. I saw pictures of Kemi holding them, her face radiant with a joy I had not seen in years, and I would be overcome with emotion. My heart ached to be with them.

When I finally arrived in Lagos, **Kemi and the twins had already been discharged from the hospital. As it happened, they had their first pediatric appointment scheduled for the day of my arrival, a perfect, God-given timing.** The sight of my wife holding our children as we waited for the doctor is a moment that is seared into my memory forever. When I finally held my son in my arms, something indescribable happened. Time stood still. All the pain, all the waiting, all the years of questions melted away in that instant. I was no longer just a husband. I was a father. A daddy.

I looked at my son, and then at my daughter, and I was overcome with a sense of awe. I thought of my own father, and the fact that I am his only son. The cultural pressure to carry on the family name had been another unspoken weight on our journey. The desire for a son was a deep, private hope I had held in my heart, a prayer I had barely dared to speak aloud. Now, here he was. God had not only answered our prayer for children; He had honored the specific, unspoken desires of our hearts. I was dancing inside. I was just super excited. *I have a son. We have a son*. It was a proud, humbling moment to know that God, in His mercy and wisdom, had entrusted me—after all these years—with these two precious lives.

The birth of our twins, Tobi and Tomi, was not just the end of a long and painful journey; it was the beginning of a new one, a journey of discovering the depth and the richness of God's faithfulness. Every aspect of their arrival felt laden with a divine significance, a sense of holy purpose that affirmed all that we had been through. This was most evident in the names we chose for them.

Once we were all together in Nigeria, we had to navigate the final logistical hurdle: getting the necessary paperwork to bring our children home to the United States. This meant dealing with embassies and government agencies, a process that can be notoriously slow and complicated. But even here, God's favor was evident. We submitted our documents to the embassy, and just a few weeks later, we were called for an interview. On December 4th, exactly one month and one day after they were born, Tobi and Tomi were officially approved. Their passports were issued, and we were cleared to go home.

The journey from Lagos to the U.S. was its own adventure. We intentionally booked a direct, eleven-hour flight, knowing that layovers with two newborns would be a nightmare. The thought of being on a plane for that long with two tiny infants was daunting. They were still so small—Tobi was about eight pounds, and Tomi was just seven. We were anxious about how they would handle the trip. But they were champions. We came prepared, our carry-on bags filled with bottles of milk, diapers, and changes of clothes. We were the last to leave the plane, taking our time to gather our small, precious family. They handled the long flight beautifully, sleeping for most of the way.

Arriving home, truly home, as a family of four was the final, surreal moment of a journey that had spanned two decades. Walking through our front door, carrying our children in their car seats, was a dream come true. The quiet halls we had walked for so many years were finally, finally filled with the sweet sounds of our babies. The silence was broken. The waiting was over.

Our first check-up with the pediatrician here in the U.S. was another moment of profound gratitude. The doctor examined them thoroughly and declared them perfectly healthy, growing beautifully. All our fears about the early delivery, the international travel—they were all laid to rest. God had protected them every step of the way. Tobi and Tomi are more than our answered prayers. They are more than the fulfillment of a dream. They are a living, breathing testimony—a declaration to the world that God still does miracles. They are not just a blessing to Kemi and me. They are a gift to the world.

Prayer Point:

Lord, we are overwhelmed with gratitude for answered prayers. Thank You for turning our deepest sorrows into our greatest joys and for redeeming every tear we have cried. In the moments when we finally hold our miracles, let the profound sense of Your faithfulness wash over us. We thank you for not only fulfilling the desires of our hearts but for honoring even the unspoken prayers we barely dared to whisper. May our lives, and the lives of our children, be a continuous song of praise to You. Amen.

Chapter 13

Lessons from the Journey

A nineteen-year journey through any valley will inevitably change you. It reshapes your landscape, redefines your horizons, and reveals a strength you never knew you possessed. My journey through the valley of infertility was long, arduous, and often heartbreaking, but it was not a wasteland. Looking back, I can see that the desolate places were where God did some of His most profound work in me. The years of waiting were not wasted years; they were years of preparation. The trials were not punishments; they were lessons in disguise. I entered this journey as a hopeful young woman, and I emerged two decades later as a different person—scarred, yes, but also stronger, more resilient, and with a deeper understanding of the God who walked with me every step of the way. These are the lessons I learned in the valley.

Lesson 1: The Power of Resilience and Consistency

This journey taught me about a strength in myself that I never knew existed: my own resilience. It also showed me the profound power of consistency. There were hundreds, if not thousands, of moments when giving up would have been the easier, more logical choice. After the fifth failed IUI, after the eleventh failed IVF cycle, after the devastating news that I could not carry my own child—giving up would have been understandable. But something inside me, a stubborn fire lit by the Holy Spirit, refused to be extinguished.

I learned that resilience isn't about not feeling pain; it's about feeling the pain and choosing to take one more step anyway. I remember one specific Tuesday morning after a failed IVF cycle. The negative result had come the day before, and the grief was a physical weight on my chest. The thought of getting out of bed, putting on professional clothes, and facing a day of meetings felt impossible. Every part of me wanted to call in sick, to hide under the covers and let the sorrow swallow me whole. But as I lay there, a quiet thought surfaced: *If I stop, the dream stops.* It wasn't a burst of inspiration, but a simple, stubborn truth. So I got up. I showered. I put on my makeup to hide the puffiness around my eyes. And I went to work.

Throughout this entire nineteen-year period, I never stopped pursuing my career. I worked full-time, earned promotions, and grew professionally, refusing to let my personal struggle derail my professional life. This consistency was a lifeline. It gave me a sense of purpose and identity outside of my infertility, which was crucial for my mental health. It reminded me that I was more than just a barren woman; I was a competent, capable professional.

Consistency in my faith was just as important, and often, just as difficult. It meant praying even when I felt like God wasn't listening. It meant showing up to church when I wanted to hide under the covers, especially on Mother's Day, when the pastor would ask all the mothers to stand and I would feel my own invisibility like a spotlight. It meant choosing to believe in His goodness, even when my circumstances looked anything but good. I remember opening my Bible with a heavy heart, my prayers feeling more like angry accusations than worship. "God, why?" I'd ask. "Why are you letting this happen?" But even in my anger, I was still turning to Him. Even in my doubt, I was still engaging with His word. This journey could have easily made me give up on God, but instead, it taught me how to grow in my faith in a way that years of ease never could have. I learned that faith isn't a feeling; it's a commitment. It's a persistent, consistent turning toward God, day after day, no matter what.

Lesson 2: Finding Purpose in the Pain

For many years, I was angry. I would look at my life and ask God, "Why is this happening to me? Why do good things seem to come so easily to other people, but my path is so hard?" It felt unfair. It felt like a punishment. I wrestled with these feelings, bringing my anger and confusion to God in my prayers. I felt like I was being punished for some unknown sin, that God was withholding His blessing from me.

Over time, and with the help of therapy, I began to see my journey from a different perspective. I started to understand that my story was not just about me. My therapist helped me reframe my thinking. She said, "Kemi, what if this isn't a punishment, but a preparation? What if God is equipping you to minister to people in a way that no one else can?" That idea was a turning point. I came to realize that I had to go through this so that I could learn from my life experiences, and in turn, help others. My pain could have a purpose. My story could become a beacon of hope for other people who were struggling in silence. It could show them that there are options, that there is still hope, that they are not alone.

This realization shifted everything for me. My journey was no longer just a personal tragedy; it was becoming a testimony. I began to understand that God wanted to use my story to encourage others, to show them His faithfulness in the midst of impossible circumstances. This is one of the most profound things I have learned: God wants us to have godly seeds, to raise children who will love and serve Him. But He also uses our journeys to plant seeds of faith in others. My story could be a seed of hope for someone else, just as other people's stories had been for me. When I later advised another couple to consider surrogacy, and they eventually had a child, their joy felt like my own. I saw the purpose in my pain in a tangible way for the first time.

Lesson 3: Handling Judgment and Criticism with Grace

Handling the judgment and criticism from others was one of the hardest parts of this journey. The hurtful comments, the unsolicited advice, the looks of pity—they were like a constant barrage of tiny arrows to the heart. I remember a woman at church who, after learning we were pursuing IVF, told me that we were interfering with God's will and that our child, if we had one, would not be a true blessing. The words were so cruel, so self-righteous, that they left me speechless and weeping in the car on the way home.

For a long time, I internalized the criticism. I believed the whispers that maybe I had done something wrong, that my faith wasn't strong enough. It was a heavy, painful burden to carry.

Therapy was instrumental in helping me navigate this. My therapist helped me understand that the judgmental comments people made were often not about me at all. She helped me realize that some people criticize or judge because they wish they had the same boldness or strength that they see in you. They see you talking openly about a difficult struggle, and it reflects their own fears and insecurities. They come to you angry or upset, but they aren't really angry at you; they have issues they are dealing with themselves. That woman from church wasn't just judging me; she was clinging to a rigid, fearful view of God that didn't allow for the mystery and wonder of His different paths.

This perspective was incredibly freeing. It allowed me to see the criticism not as an attack on my character, but as a reflection of someone else's pain. It didn't make the words hurt any less, but it did help me to not let them take root in my heart. I learned to handle these situations with grace, to smile and thank them for their "concern," while privately giving their words to God and refusing to let them define me. I realized I cannot live other people's dreams or meet their expectations. I can only live my life, the one God has given me.

Lesson 4: The Unbreakable Strength of Community

This journey taught me that community support is not just a nice idea; it is a vital, non-negotiable lifeline. There is absolutely no way I could have survived this journey without the incredible support of my friends and family. They were my big support, my prayer warriors, my encouragers.

My cousins, my friends, my church family—they were the ones who stood in the gap for me when I was too weak to stand for myself. They were the ones who didn't offer easy answers, but simply sat with me in my grief. I thank God for them. They never insulted me or gave me looks of pity; they were just a constant source of encouragement. After the devastating encounter in May 2012, when a woman questioned my spirit and my grief over my mother's recent passing was still so raw, it was my friends who rallied around me. They called, they texted, they showed up at my house with food and hugs. They didn't try to explain away the woman's cruelty; they just validated my pain and reminded me of God's truth. They played a huge role in where I am today, because they created a safe space where I could be open and vulnerable without fear of judgment.

Accepting their help, especially the financial help for the surrogacy, was a huge lesson in humility for me. My first instinct was to say no. I was embarrassed and ashamed that we couldn't do it on our own. But I remembered what my therapist had said about allowing others the blessing of giving. When my husband and I finally agreed to let our community help, it was one of the most beautiful and humbling experiences of our lives. It was the body of Christ in action, living out the command to bear one another's burdens.

We also learned the importance of being intentional about our community. We had to create boundaries and learn to be selective about who we shared the intimate details of our journey with. We couldn't share our hopes and fears with those who would meet them with judgment or negativity. We had to cultivate a small, trusted circle of supporters who would cover us in prayer and speak life over us. This taught us that while we are called to be in community, we are also called to be wise about who we allow to have a voice in our lives.

Lesson 5: A New Relationship with Faith and Motherhood

This journey has completely redefined what faith means to me. I used to think of faith as believing for a specific outcome. Now, I understand that faith is trusting in the character of God, regardless of the outcome. My journey was one of walking by faith, even when I couldn't see how it was going to happen. I wasn't sure if I would become a mother by getting pregnant myself, or through adoption, or through a surrogate. For a long time, surrogacy wasn't even on my radar. But I knew, one way or the other, that I was going to be a mother. I held on to that belief, that promise, and I was willing to explore whatever path God opened up for me. When the option of carrying a pregnancy myself was taken away, I looked at the embryos we had preserved and knew that surrogacy was the next step of faith God was calling me to.

This journey also changed my relationship with my body. For years, I saw my body as a failure, a source of shame and disappointment. I was angry at it for not doing what it was "supposed" to do. But through this process, and especially through therapy, I learned to have compassion for my body. I began to see it not as a failure, but as a body that had endured so much—multiple surgeries, years of powerful hormones, the physical toll of grief and stress. I learned to thank it for its resilience, for carrying me through the fight. This shift in perspective was profoundly healing.

And finally, becoming a mother has changed me in beautiful ways. It has made me more patient. When you have waited nineteen years for something, you learn a thing or two about patience! It has made me more loving and more compassionate. It has helped me to see people beyond their flaws and to understand that everyone is going to through their own private struggles. It has taught me a new level of consistency and selflessness that I could have never understood before. Every sleepless night, every diaper change, every moment spent comforting a crying child is a gift, a privilege I do not take for granted.

This journey has taught me to remain consistent and to never give up. There is always light at the end of the tunnel. It may not be the outcome you expected, but God's plan is always better than our own. He is a God of miracles, and He is still writing beautiful stories. Our story is a testament to that, and it is our prayer that it will be a source of hope and encouragement for all who read it.

Prayer Point:

Father, we thank You not just for the destination, but for the lessons learned in the valley. We praise You for the resilience, strength, and deeper faith that can only be forged in the fire of waiting. We ask that you redeem our pain for a purpose. May the story of our struggle become a

beacon of hope for others, a testament to Your unwavering faithfulness. Amen.

Chapter 14
Breaking the Silence

Our journey did not end when we brought our children home. In many ways, that was the beginning of a new and unexpected chapter: the chapter of our testimony. The private, nineteen-year battle had become a public story of God's faithfulness, and we quickly learned that sharing our story was not just a desire, but a responsibility. It has been a profound privilege to walk with others on their own journeys, to see our story, which was born from so much private pain, become a lifeline for someone else. We have had the honor of sitting with two other couples, holding their hands as they made the brave decision to pursue surrogacy because of what God did for us. Seeing their joy, holding their children, and knowing that our pain had a purpose beyond our own family has been one of the most rewarding experiences of my life. It confirmed what I had begun to learn in the valley: God does not waste our suffering. He truly uses it to create rivers in the desert for others to find their way. Our willingness to be vulnerable has allowed others who were battling in the silence, just as we once had, to find a path forward, and for that, I am eternally grateful.

I remember one afternoon, sitting in our living room with the first couple. Our own twins were toddlers then, making a joyful mess in the corner, a constant, beautiful reminder of God's faithfulness. This couple, dear friends of ours, sat on the couch, their shoulders heavy with the weight of their own years of failed treatments. The wife looked at me, her eyes filled with a familiar mixture of hope and terror, and asked, "But weren't you scared? Scared of it not working, scared of the distance, scared of what people would say?" I took a deep breath and told her the absolute truth. "Terrified," I said. "Every single day. But the fear of staying in the same place of silent pain finally became greater than the fear of stepping out into the unknown." We talked for hours, not just about the logistics and the costs, but about the spiritual warfare, the emotional toll, and the incredible peace that comes with finally surrendering to a path you know God has opened. When their own beautiful baby girl was born, and they placed her in my arms, I wept. It was as if I was looking at a tangible piece of my own answered prayer, a living continuation of our story.

My response today to questions or even negative comments about surrogacy is very different from what it would have been years ago. The old me, the one still raw from years of judgment, would have been hurt, defensive, and quick to shut down. I would have felt the need to justify my choices, to prove the validity of my motherhood. Now, by the grace of God and the healing that has taken place in my heart, I see it as an opportunity for ministry. When someone makes a negative comment, my first response is to pray silently for wisdom and grace. I remind myself that their words are often rooted in fear or misinformation, not malice. Outwardly, I usually start with a smile. I've learned that a gentle demeanor can disarm a critical spirit. I thank them for their concern, which often takes them by surprise, and then I try to lovingly and patiently educate people. I'll say something like, "I understand why it might seem strange or different, but for us, it was a medical necessity, just like a kidney transplant would be for someone whose kidneys have failed." By framing it in a medical context they can understand, it often shifts their perspective from one of moral judgment to one of human compassion.

I can almost picture the conversation. A well-meaning church aunty might say, "Ah, Kemi, but is that God's way? Shouldn't you just have waited for God to open your womb?" Instead of bristling, I can now say, "Aunty, we waited for nineteen years. We prayed, we fasted, and we believed. And then, we believe God opened a different door. He gave doctors wisdom, just as He gave Solomon wisdom. For us, this was His way." I've learned that people's reactions are often a reflection of their own rigid theological boxes. They simply haven't considered that God can work in ways they haven't seen before. It's no longer about defending my choices; it's about sharing God's faithfulness in a way they may have never considered. In the Nigerian community, the idea of another woman carrying your child can feel so foreign, but when I explain that our children are biologically ours, and that this woman was a "helper," an answer to prayer, something clicks for them. It's a slow process, but it is changing the conversation, one person at a time.

What I want people in my community to understand about fertility treatments is that pursuing them is not a failure of faith; for many of us, it is an act of profound faith. It is taking the little we have—our hope, our resources, our courage—and placing it in the hands of God, asking Him to bless it through the means He has made available. We must stop seeing science as the opposite of God. God is the author of all knowledge, the creator of the human mind that develops these medical marvels. Why would we believe He is not also in the science that helps create families? While cultural opinions will always shift and sway, God's word must always be the compass. These treatments are simply a path to fulfilling God's promise of family for those who cannot get there on their own. I often think back to that "sisterhood of unspoken sorrow" I felt in the waiting rooms, and my prayer is that our community can become a place of open support, not silent judgment.

To the couples who are still waiting, who feel like you are in the trenches of a long and brutal war, my message is this: do not give up. Resilience and consistency are your greatest weapons. I know you are weary. I know the thought of another cycle, another appointment, another two-week wait feels impossible. But you are stronger than you know. Be consistent in your pursuit and be willing to explore every option God places before you. And lean on your community. Find those friends who will pray for you when you don't have the strength to pray for yourself, because you will need them. On the days when my own faith felt like a flickering candle, I would call my friend Abbey. I wouldn't even have to say anything; she could hear the exhaustion in my silence. And she would just begin to pray, her strong, unwavering faith becoming a shield around my own. That is the power of community. It is not just about casseroles and condolences; it is about spiritually holding up each other's arms in the midst of the battle.

I am particularly passionate about changing the conversation about infertility in the Black community. We must break the silence that has surrounded this topic for too long. My hope is to normalize the conversation, to dismantle the stigma by sharing our stories. Our journeys are not a mark of failure; they are a testament to our profound faith. As a practical first step for any couple considering surrogacy, I have three pieces of advice. First, acknowledge that it is staggeringly expensive, and begin planning and saving with intention. My husband and I created a "baby fund" years before we even knew what path we would take. Every extra dollar, every bonus, every small sacrifice went into that account. It was an act of faith, preparing for a miracle we could not yet see. Second, find a supportive community and a Christian therapist; these were vital to our journey. A therapist helps you unpack the trauma, and a community helps you carry the burden. Third, prepare your hearts. While the physical part of the journey may be over for you, the emotional one continues in a new and beautiful way.

As we share our story, we are careful to balance it with protecting our children's privacy. This is our testimony, not theirs. We focus on our journey of faith, not the intimate details of their lives. This book is a testament to God's faithfulness, a story for them to read when they're older so they can fully understand the miraculous meaning behind their names: Tobi and Tomi, Joshua and Hannah. It is their spiritual heritage, a permanent record of the prayers that were answered to bring them into this world.

So, what does "faith prevailed" mean to me now? It does not mean that because we had faith, we got the outcome we wanted. It means that our faith, in and of itself, *survived*. It prevailed over the immense cultural pressure that told me I was less of a woman. It prevailed over the crippling financial strain that threatened to break us. It prevailed over every single one of the repeated medical failures that declared my body a barren wasteland. The victory was not the arrival of our children; the children are the extravagant evidence of God's grace. The victory was won in the waiting. It was won in the quiet moments of choosing to trust God one more time, when every human reason told me to give up.

Prayer Point:

Lord, thank You for the privilege of our testimony. Give us the courage to break the silence and share our story with grace and boldness, not for our own glory, but for Yours. Use our words to dismantle stigma, to offer hope, and to be a lifeline for others who are battling in silence. May our journey continue to be a river in the desert for all who need to find their way. Amen.

Conclusion

If I could sit across from you right now, a couple in year ten of your journey, your hearts aching with that familiar, weary pain, the first thing I would do is just look at you and say, "**I see you**." I see the weariness in your eyes, the forced smiles, the **fragile hope** you are so afraid to cling to. I want you to know that **everything you are feeling is valid**. I remember what year ten felt like. It was a strange, lonely place, a landscape of quiet grief punctuated by the loud joy of everyone else's life. I remember sitting at a baby shower around that time, holding a beautifully wrapped gift, my smile feeling like a mask that was about to crack. I watched the mother-to-be, radiant and full of life, open onesies and tiny shoes, and a voice in my head whispered, *This will never be you.* I had to physically excuse myself and go to the bathroom, locking the door behind me just to breathe, to push back the tears that were threatening to spill over. That is the weary pain I'm talking about. It's the pain of a thousand paper cuts, of a hope that has been deferred for so long it has made your heart sick. It's the pain of feeling invisible in a world that is so focused on family. So please, hear me when I say this: you are not crazy, you are not faithless, and you are not alone.

Then, after sitting with you in that space of honesty, I would gently take your hands and say, "**Your story is not over. The page you are on right now... is not the final chapter.**" I know it feels like it, but **God is the author of the most beautiful stories**, and **delay is not denial**.

I know the financial struggle of this journey is immense. For **couples who can't afford treatments**, the cost can feel like a cruel joke. My encouragement to you is to pair your faith with action. Begin **planning and saving**, and trust that **God will provide. It's not always easy, but God will provide.** But I want to be practical here. This isn't just about praying for money to fall from the sky. It's about being wise stewards of what you have and creating a plan. Sit down together and create a "miracle budget." Look at every single expense and ask, "Is this more important than our dream?" It might mean forgoing vacations for a few years, driving an older car, or cutting back on eating out. It might mean taking on a side job. My husband and I did all of those things. It wasn't a punishment; it was an investment in our future. And as you are faithful with the practical steps, pray with specificity. Pray for God to open doors of provision, to give you creative ideas, and to bless the work of your hands. Your faith will grow not just in the waiting, but in the working.

I also know that sometimes, the greatest pain comes from our own families when they **don't support our journey**. This is where you must remember that while you are called to honor your family, your primary covenant is to God and to your spouse. **God's Word must always be the compass.** Build your own **circle of godly, wise friends** who will be your **lifeline**, who will protect you from harmful conversations, just as my husband did for me. I can imagine the conversation with a well-meaning but hurtful relative. They might say, "You are spending all this money on doctors? Why don't you just trust God?" A loving but firm response could be, "We are trusting God. And we believe He is the one who has given us the wisdom to seek help through the doctors He has equipped. We would love for you to pray with us on this path." You do not have to defend your choices, but you can, and should, defend your boundaries.

When people **remember my story**, I hope they remember the journey, not just the outcome. I hope they see that faith can survive doubt, pain, loss, and grief. The children are not the victory, but the **extravagant evidence** of a victory that was won in the waiting.

And to my own children, **Tobi and Tomi**, when you read this book one day, I hope you see it as your **spiritual heritage**. I hope you see that this is not a story of my pain, but a story of God's profound faithfulness to our family, a legacy of resilience for your own lives. I want you to understand the meaning behind your names—that God is a Great King, and that His blessings are always sufficient.

This book is the story of how we met you, a spiritual roadmap that I pray will guide you back to the heart of a Father who loved you even before we did.

My **final message** to anyone reading this book is simple: your story is not over. God is still writing. I pray a blessing of peace and strength over you right now, that you would feel the tangible presence of a God who sees you, who loves you, and who is faithful to complete the good work He has started in you.

My husband's final thoughts are a perfect way to end this book on a note of shared triumph and a call to action. As a man in our community, he faced his own unique set of pressures, and his perspective is vital. His message to other husbands is a powerful charge to lead with love, humility, and unwavering faith. I've learned that **science and faith are not enemies**, and his final words are a beautiful testament to the God who works in all things to fulfill His promises.

My Husband's Final Thoughts: Faith, Pressure, and the Promise Fulfilled

The Hardest Part: "Watching my wife go through the rollercoaster of disappointments, failed treatments, and emotional strain was heartbreaking. What made it worse was the cultural expectation—especially within the Yoruba community—that infertility is solely a woman's issue. The silence, the blame, the judgment... all of it weighed heavily on us."

Handling Cultural Pressure: "In Yoruba culture, if a couple has no children, the woman is typically blamed first. As a man, it would've been easy to hide behind that narrative. But love doesn't shift blame; it shares burdens. What preserved our marriage was our love for God, and for each other. I had to lead with humility and courage—sometimes confronting family with grace, protecting my wife from harmful conversations, and choosing biblical truth over cultural opinion. Culture will always have an opinion, but God's Word must always be the compass."

Supporting My Wife: "I made a conscious decision early on: with or without children, our marriage would succeed. That decision became our anchor. I reminded her of that often. We built a circle of godly, wise friends who kept us grounded. And above all, we stayed committed to God in prayer, worship, and devotion. That was our oxygen."

A Message to Other Husbands: "Stay the course. Infertility will test your faith, your love, and your commitment. There were days I felt like walking away—but I chose to stay, to trust God, and to love my wife unconditionally. Be accountable—to God, to a mentor, to your community. Don't walk alone. And never forget: science and faith are not enemies. God can and does use medical processes to fulfill His promises. Keep your heart open and your eyes on Him."

Becoming a Father After 21 Years: "When I first held our twins, I was in awe of what God had done. It wasn't just the joy of becoming a father—it was the weight of every prayer, every disappointment, every ounce of hope fulfilled. I felt like I was holding God's faithfulness. After 21 years, I finally heard it: 'Daddy.' That single word erased decades of pain. God is faithful. Always."

Scriptural References

Isaiah 40:31: "But those who trust in the Lord will find new strength. They will soar high on wings like eagles. They will run and not grow weary. They will walk and not faint."

Psalm 37:4-5: "Take delight in the Lord, and he will give you your heart's desires. Commit everything you do to the Lord. Trust him, and he will help you."

Lamentations 3:22-23: "The faithful love of the Lord never ends! His mercies never cease. Great is his faithfulness; his mercies begin afresh each morning."

Romans 8:28: "And we know that God causes everything to work together for the good of those who love God and are called according to his purpose for them."

Psalm 127:3: "Children are a gift from the Lord; they are a reward from him."

Genesis 1:28: "Then God blessed them and said, 'Be fruitful and multiply. Fill the earth and govern it. Reign over the fish in the sea, the birds in the sky, and all the animals that scurry along the ground.'"

Exodus 23:26: "There will be no miscarriages or infertility in your land, and I will give you long, full lives."

Scripture and Reflection

Here are some scriptures to meditate on as you navigate your journey:

- **Romans 5:3-5 (NIV)**"...suffering produces perseverance; perseverance, character; and character, hope. And hope does not put us to shame..."

- **Ecclesiastes 3:11 (NLT)**"Yet God has made everything beautiful for its own time..."

- **James 1:12 (NIV)**"Blessed is the one who perseveres under trial because, having stood the test, that person will receive the crown of life..."

For Reflection or Couples Discussion

This journey can be isolating, not just from the world, but sometimes from each other. Use these questions as a starting point for conversation—to connect, to understand, and to strengthen your bond as you walk this path together.

1. What cultural pressures have impacted your view of infertility, and how can you replace them with biblical truth?

2. As a husband, what does it mean to "take the lead with humility" in protecting and honoring your wife?

3. How do you support each other emotionally and spiritually in seasons of disappointment?

4. What boundaries have you set—or need to set—with family or community regarding your fertility journey?

5. Where do you see the hand of God working in your story, even if the answer hasn't come yet?

Glossary

Chemical Pregnancy

A very early miscarriage, typically occurring within the first five weeks of pregnancy, before an embryo can be seen on an ultrasound. These are often caused by chromosomal abnormalities.

Fallopian Tubes

The reproductive organs that transport eggs from the ovaries to the uterus. Their removal makes natural pregnancy extremely unlikely.

Fibroids

Non-cancerous, solid growths that develop on the wall of the uterus, often requiring medical intervention for removal if they cause symptoms or complications.

Frozen Embryos

Embryos created through in vitro fertilization (IVF) that are cryopreserved (frozen at a very low temperature) for future use. This allows for subsequent pregnancies without the need for another full IVF cycle.

Gestational Carrier

A woman who carries and delivers a baby for another person or couple. She has no genetic relationship to the child she carries, as the embryo is created via in vitro fertilization (IVF) using the intended parents' or donors' genetic material and then implanted into her uterus. (This differs from a traditional surrogate, who uses her own egg and is biologically related to the child.)

IUI (Intrauterine Insemination)

A fertility treatment that involves the direct placement of sperm into a woman's uterus to facilitate fertilization.

IVF (In Vitro Fertilization)

A complex series of procedures used to assist with fertility, prevent genetic problems, and aid in the conception of a child. During IVF, mature eggs are retrieved from the ovaries and fertilized by sperm in a laboratory setting.

Ovarian Cysts

Fluid-filled sacs or growths that develop on or within the ovaries. While often benign, they can cause health complications if they become too large, rupture, or cause pain.

Surrogacy

An arrangement, often supported by a legal agreement, whereby a woman agrees to bear a child for another person or people, who will become the child's parent(s) after birth. This can be done through traditional surrogacy (where the surrogate is the biological mother) or gestational surrogacy (see Gestational Carrier).

Uterus

A hollow, pear-shaped organ located in a woman's pelvis where a fetus develops and grows during pregnancy. Also referred to as the womb.

www.ingramcontent.com/pod-product-compliance
Lightning Source LLC
Chambersburg PA
CBHW071327130626
46556CB00004B/1779